To Kathy Barton
(Angela Lynn Roles, birthname)

Facing Teenage Pregnancy

A Handbook for the Pregnant Teen

Third Edition

Patricia Roles, MSW

CWLA Press

CWLA Press is an imprint of the Child Welfare League of America. The Child Welfare League of America is the nation's oldest and largest membership-based child welfare organization. We are committed to engaging people everywhere in promoting the well-being of children, youth, and their families, and protecting every child from harm.

Child Welfare League of America, Inc.
440 First Street, NW, Third Floor, Washington, DC 20001-2085
E-mail: books@cwla.org

Current Printing (last digit)
10 9 8 7 6 5 4 3 2 1

Printed in the United States of America

ISBN 10: 1-58760-041-2

ISBN 13: 978-1-58760-041-8

Library of Congress Cataloging-in-Publication Data

Roles, Patricia.
 Facing teenage pregnancy : a handbook for the pregnant teen / Patricia Roles.-- 3rd ed.
    p. cm.
 ISBN 1-58760-041-2 (alk. paper)
 1. Teenage pregnancy--Psychological aspects. 2. Teenage mothers. 3. Pregnancy, Unwanted--Decision making. I. Child Welfare League of America. II. Title.

HQ759.4.R64 2005
306.874'3--dc22

2005002283

Contents

Acknowledgments

I thank my family, friends, and colleagues who encouraged and supported me while I was writing this book. My appreciation is extended to those at Children's Hospital in Vancouver, who made my leave of absence possible so that I might complete this project, and to Claire Thomson, who assisted me with many practical matters. I offer special thanks to Debbie, Jon, Lori, Bruce, Linda, and Suzanne for generously sharing their personal experiences with me and adding the sensitivity that makes the people in this book realizable. I am grateful to Stephen Parrish, who recognized the need for this publication and who, with the skillful editing provided by Mrs. Virginia Bennet, made it a reality.

Introduction

In picking up this book, you are taking the first step toward finding the help you need. In the end, you will realize that you have found a great part of that help within yourself and from your own strength.

In 1969, when I thought that I must have been the only teenager who had ever become pregnant, I might have benefited from a book that addressed my troubles. I felt lost and alone. There was nobody with whom I could talk, nobody who had faced what I was facing. I wondered if anyone would understand my problem if I told them about it. It would have helped me to have known that other girls were in the same predicament. I might have been able to learn from them how to prepare myself for the consequences of my pregnancy. I might have learned from them that help was available.

Each of us believes, "It can't happen to me." So did I. Perhaps you are thinking now as I thought in 1969: How could I have prepared for something I did not think would happen to me? Perhaps you are as confused as I was.

This book is based on the premise that teenage pregnancies will continue to occur. It is, therefore, designed as an aid to those girls who find themselves faced with the dilemma of being unmarried, teenaged, pregnant, and in need of learning how to cope with what lies ahead for them. Rather than denying that the problem exists and closing our eyes to it in the hope that it will go away, it is time we tried to help those who have to live through the experience. Although we might like to believe that our moral values have changed substantially since 1969, we are compelled to recognize that the unmarried pregnant teenager is still subject to social pressures.

Teenage pregnancy is not only a social issue but also a personal problem. Teenage girls unintentionally become pregnant despite the prevailing open discussion of sexual matters in our society. They are not so sophisticated as we would like to believe and are still subject to misinformation. We should always stress prevention, especially in trying to educate younger teenage girls. We also need to support those girls who are presently in need of help.

Although each young girl's situation is unique, some problems are common to all unmarried teenagers facing an unwanted pregnancy and the decisions they have to make because of it. The world may seem to be caving in when pregnancy is confirmed. But every crisis is also an opportunity through which we can learn and grow and survive. It may be impossible for you to believe now that this experience may enrich rather than destroy your life, but we grow the most and learn the best when change and pain enter our lives.

I vividly remember that my social worker told me that I would learn something from my pregnancy. At the time, I failed to see what it could possibly be. Later on, her words made sense to me, and I valued her assurances because they helped me on the way to understanding the positive elements underlying my negative turmoil. Keep in mind as you read this book that you can learn something special from this crisis in your life. You can become more aware of yourself and of others. This understanding may grow and deepen your sensitivity to others. You need not lower your aspirations nor abandon your goals. Your life is not ruined. You can look forward to fulfilling years afterward.

I chose to place my baby for adoption. It felt like the only choice for me at the time. Abortion was not easily accessible back then. I also waited too long to tell anyone, so lost this as an option.

Perhaps you are an unmarried pregnant girl and are as yet undecided whether to offer your baby for adoption. Or perhaps you have already decided on another course. You should be aware that this book is not an endorsement of any one decision as a best one but only a presentation of my own perspective along with some experiences for teenagers who chose other alternatives. My aim is to aid you in making your own decision and in coping with the consequences of your decision and putting your life back together afterwards. No option is easy.

I am sharing with you my own experience of teenage pregnancy and my subsequent education and career. I obtained a master's degree in social work and now work in a hospital for children and adolescents. I hope that my dual perspective will benefit not only you, the teenager, but also the professionals, family, and friends who are in a position to offer support to you. Family and friends are in a vulnerable position. They can play a supportive role but may in turn be affected by your situation and may themselves need support. This book may help you when you are burdened with an unwanted pregnancy and wondering what to do next. It is not a list of tips on how to cope with your problems, but in reading about the initial shock I felt on learning that I was pregnant and about how I subsequently coped with it, you may be assisted in exploring your own situation more fully.

Although this book is primarily addressed to the pregnant teenager and to the significant people in her life, it may prove useful to the adopted teenager who is troubled by thoughts about being adopted. She may gain an awareness and an understanding of her birthmother's decision to place her for adoption.

First and foremost, every pregnant girl needs to know that she is okay. The strength that comes from appreciating yourself is your key to coping with any problems you may have, including your pregnancy. Strong knowledge of your own worthiness will help you withstand social pressures and will increase your chances of making your experience a gain rather than a loss. Do not resign yourself to being devastated by events. Envision your predicament and the course you take as another part of living designed to help you grow into a better person.

I hope that this book may inspire you. Being pregnant doesn't have to make you a loser, a failure, or even a school dropout. It is a condition demanding your determination to direct your energy toward making your experience productive while maintaining your sense of personal dignity.

Chapter 1

How It All Begins

How could I have wanted more at this point in my life? Everything seemed to be about right. I had a middle-class happy family. I did not lack for friends. I lived in a small town and was a good student, had career ambitions, a steady boyfriend, and all the rest. At the youthful age of 15, I was just getting into the excitement of learning about the sexual aspects of male/female relationships. But I was soon to discover something that would turn my immediate, safe world inside out and make a lasting impression on the years to come: I was to find out that I was pregnant.

After I missed my first period, I kept hoping as each day went by that it would come soon, but it didn't. Being too embarrassed to take a urine sample for a pregnancy test, I asked my boyfriend to take it to the pharmacy. He received the bad news and then had to tell me. We both sat in shock and disbelief, but at least we were together.

If you are reading this book, you may have already learned that you are pregnant. If you do not yet know whether you are or are not, be sure to go to a store or pharmacy and obtain a home-testing kit to determine what you are probably wondering about. You may be worrying needlessly, but it is better to know what you are dealing with than it is to go on hoping it might go away on its own. Pregnancy tests with instructions are available on the shelf at the pharmacy, and you can discover whether you are pregnant without any shame. You can test for pregnancy as soon as 6 to 12 days after ovulation. For more accurate results, however, it is best to wait one week after the first day of your missed period. Follow the instructions on the test kit. A test taken too soon may give you a false result: It could read negative when in fact you are pregnant. If the test proves positive, you should immediately have a medical checkup. This entails an internal examination in which the physician inserts two fingers into your vagina to determine whether your uterus has begun to expand.

Time is a vital element. In waiting to see whether you miss a second period, you may lose valuable time and may wait too long for an abortion to be safe. Some girls grasp at other causes for a late period and hope that they are not pregnant.

Shock

This couldn't have happened to me. Why me? Of course this only happened to bad or promiscuous girls, and I was not that kind of girl. I naturally didn't see myself as either bad or promiscuous, so it had to be impossible that I was pregnant. I must have been dreaming, and I would wake up soon.

Perhaps you, too, have been caught up in the excitement of new sexual feelings and have had sex with someone. And perhaps you have actually considered that it might happen, that you might become pregnant. But until you actually do become pregnant, you cannot be fully aware of all the implications of pregnancy.

A flood of contradictory feelings during the initial shock of discovery is to be expected when you are taken by surprise. You cannot prepare for what you have never expected to happen, especially if you have taken birth control precautions, as I had. Who would expect birth control to fail? You may feel fear, shame, anger, guilt, sadness, frustration, despair, and self-pity. You may feel trapped, cornered, desperate—as though you have no way out. You may not be ready to cope with the reality of your situation. It takes time to digest the thought that it is really happening, and is happening to you. You may convince yourself that even if it is frightening now, things will get better later. And so you may settle into the comfort of disbelief.

Until now, you may not have had a problem so grave as pregnancy to deal with. But now you have no choice. You must pull yourself together and try your best to deal with your problem. It will seem as though you have been thrust overnight into an adult world and have adult decisions to make before your time. This is a quick jump into adulthood, so let an adult be the shoulder you lean on. You will need someone. It is not a sign of weakness to seek help. It is a sign of strength. We all need help at some time in our lives.

Talk to someone right away. Your parents would be the best helpers. If you feel you cannot tell them yet, perhaps you could tell another family member, friend, teacher, or adult. If not, there are crisis phone lines, school counselors, teen clinics, or your family doctor. You need to find someone to help you with this initial crisis.

Denial

In the beginning, you may reject the fact of your pregnancy, and then you may gradually deny it altogether. You may try to put off the inevitable for as long as possible, but this denial is helpful for only a short while. Denial affords you some essential time for sorting out your thoughts and preparing yourself to deal with the issues you face so that you may adjust to the fact that you are pregnant.

Before you are reconciled to the reality of your condition and your ability to cope with it, you may think of suicide. You may feel desperate for any way out. It may seem as though there is no way out, because your mind is clouded and confused and you cannot see clearly. But remember that you are still your original self. And you are still a worthwhile person. Remember that there are people who care about you.

Postpone making any decisions until your thoughts and feelings are less chaotic. And they will be. Talking with your boyfriend, a close friend, or an adult at this time my help you to sort out your feelings and dispel your confusion. Talking with your family may be as yet too overwhelming an experience, because you may fear your parents' reaction. But the chances are that they would only try to help you in any way they know how.

You cannot begin to cope with your pregnancy until after you have recovered from the shock of realization and have ceased to deny the reality of your pregnancy. Denying it is only a temporary crutch, and until you begin to accept it, you cannot begin to consider the options open to you. You have the right to choose an alternative to pregnancy, and support is available to you, whatever course you choose to follow. If denial persists too long, an abortion may not be possible. An abortion performed early in your pregnancy is less complicated than one performed later in the pregnancy. If you put off accepting that you are pregnant, it may be too late for an abortion, should you have wanted to make that choice. Denial not only diminishes the number of choices open to you but also denies you the prenatal care necessary for your own health as well as for your baby's health, should you decide to carry the baby to term.

My own semi-denial, or living out a fantasy, lasted six months before I was able to accept my predicament and begin to face it. By then I had lost the option of abortion. Perhaps you are wondering who I am to talk about the need for early acceptance. I can only say hindsight is wonderful. I know how easy it is to fool yourself into thinking that your growing stomach will go away, as if by magic or natural miscarriage.

The old wives' tale remedies were of no avail to me. Mustard baths and castor oil had no effect on my pregnancy. They were not only a waste of time, but they were also a source of disappointment. My nose still turns up at the smell of castor oil.

In 1969, I had little to lose by denying everything, because it was not so easy then to get an abortion. From Canada, one had to go to New York with a lot of money or else seek a backstreet abortion—illegal, crude, and unsafe. Some girls who did not have the money to go to New York were unfortunately desperate enough to submit to those crude abortions, and some girls died from them. Today we are fortunate that abortions are performed in hospitals and clinics under safe conditions in sterile surroundings.

Facing the Facts

After having run scared for more than five months and having kept my secret, I slowly began to accept the truth. It had become a physical impossibility to keep my condition hidden any longer from those around me. In looking back, I find it hard to believe that my parents still had not realized that I was pregnant after almost six months. I had endured teasing about getting fat that had brought me to the brink of tears. I am sure now that my parents must have wondered why I was so overly sensitive. My cover-up had gone so far as faking menstrual periods by discarding sanitary napkins so that Mom wouldn't suspect anything or question me. I had feared that I might have broken down and cried if she had asked me anything at all.

You can imagine the energy, fear, and determination I had needed to hide my pregnancy. My relief in abandoning the pretense was as intense as the fear that had prompted it. But it was not until I revealed my pregnancy that I was able to begin facing up to it. It was then that I began to regain my sanity. It was then that I began to direct my energy and my determination toward making positive plans to deal with the months ahead.

In delaying the telling for so long, I had denied myself and my baby proper medical care. Two weeks after confessing my condition, I was hospitalized with toxemia. Although my illness was a setback attributable to my neglect of myself and my baby, I benefited by being in the hospital. I was directly faced with the fact of pregnancy. Doctors and nurses checked for the baby's heartbeat, and I had my first visit from a social worker. Because of the toxemia, I had to go on a salt-free diet and rest more than I wanted. A healthy pregnancy is an easier pregnancy, and it also eases your guilt to know that you have done your best to see that your baby receives proper medical attention.

Before you accept your pregnancy, you may do a lot of crying and have many uncomfortable feelings. Perhaps you are thinking that this was not one of the goals you would have set for yourself. There are many fears about facing the facts. You may fear rejection by your family, friends, or boyfriend. You may dread the responsibility of being a mother. You may fear the possible loss of a year at school. You may feel that your pregnancy will interfere with relationships or with marriage. You may wonder whether you will be able to bring yourself to give your baby up for adoption. You may be troubled by abortion as being morally wrong. You may feel that you are being punished for something. Your thoughts are confused, and you may wonder how to find help.

But once you bring the issue into the open, you put it into perspective. People can then reach out and help you; you are no longer all alone. A certain peace of mind evolves, a peace that frees you to explore orderly alternatives to the confusion you have been suffering. You are able to make realistic and practical decisions and to impose an order of your own choice on the events of your future life.

Whatever you choose, it won't be easy. There is no easy answer and no easy choice open to the pregnant teenager. But knowing what you plan to do helps you to clear up the chaos. The unknown increases your sense of turmoil. In knowing, you will no longer feel that your head is spinning. As your thoughts come less rapidly and chaotically, you will find room to breathe.

Life is a series of changes and adaptations. It never stands still or stays the same. Change may come too suddenly or too often for you, spinning you in circles. But change is also productive and provides you with stimulation and growth. With only stability, you get bored; with only change, you get overwhelmed. So you need a balance between stability and change.

Pregnancy precipitates radical changes in many areas of your life, now and later on. Try to see where you can find some stability and order right now to balance the heavy stress of the news of your pregnancy. You need to restore that delicate balance, the mix of change and order, as in all the significant life events, such as changing schools, leaving home, getting married, losing or beginning a job, or retiring. The balance won't be exactly the same as before. Things have changed; it will be a new balance.

Alternatives

By now you have searched every avenue for answers and are accepting the facts. Now you are forced to think about what your alternatives are. This means finding out as much as you can about the options available to you, approaching resource people, asking questions, looking at both the immediate and the long-term consequences of those options, and eventually deciding on a course of action. Keep your eyes open for help along the way.

You have four basic alternatives: marriage or living together, adoption, keeping your baby as a single parent, and abortion. We shall explore these alternatives in some detail here and in subsequent chapters. Each one has its benefits and challenges. No alternative is easy.

Marriage

Marriage is obviously the most socially acceptable alternative, but is unfortunately a further change in itself. Even positive changes call for adaptation. You will need to get used to being a wife or partner and mother all at once, sort out what to do about school, and leave home. You would likely have a teenage husband or partner facing just as many changes in having to become a father before he is really ready. He may still be in school and have no secure job. He may be unable to support a family until he completes school. As he will be going through changes similar to those you are going through, he too will be under stress. Consequently, he might be wrapped up in his own struggle to adapt and unable to meet your needs.

It may seem romantic. It may be good to feel that you are not alone, but unless marriage was already in your immediate plans before your pregnancy, you should question why you now feel like getting married. Is it for social acceptance, is it a way out, or is it what you would really choose for your life right now?

If the marriage or living together does not work out because of all these pressures, you would be left with the stress of separation added to your responsibilities as a single parent to provide support for yourself and your baby. Marrying to escape an already difficult situation could bring you an even more complex set of problems. Think through your reasons for marrying carefully and determine whether pressure is coming from anyone to take this socially acceptable route or whether it is what you really want.

Committing to a relationship through marriage or a common-law union can be a joyous, exciting time. If this is the case for you, having two parents for your baby is a blessing. It is not a quick fix, however, as relationships take hard work, maturity, and commitment.

Adoption

After having a fetus growing inside you for nine months, you cannot deny that an attachment is formed. The attachment grows as you feel the life inside you grow and move. In going to term, you have gone through a lot together with your baby, so you need to prepare yourself for the feelings of loss when you give your baby up for adoption. The sense of loss is keener after giving birth than it is in undergoing abortion before an attachment is formed. The loss is heightened by going through labor pains without the joy that makes it all seem worthwhile in a wanted pregnancy. This leaves you feeling empty and futile. You can expect to feel the sense of loss and the weight of sadness at leaving your baby behind as you walk out through the hospital doors. For me, this was the hardest part.

It is common to feel downcast around the anniversary of the birth of your child. Having another baby will not replace the lost one. The loss is painful. Adoption relinquishment does not end when you sign adoption papers. The effect is lifelong.

But after looking at these feelings, which are your emotional side, you must always keep in touch with your intellectual side. This intellectual side reminds you that you have chosen a course you considered best for your baby as well as best for yourself in the long run. You want your child to have the best.

Fewer babies are being placed for adoption than ever before. This means that adopting couples may wait more than five years to adopt a child. Hopefully, the positive side of this is that adoptive parents who are eager for children will provide caring homes. There are no guarantees in life, however, and no way of ensuring the quality of life for your child in an adoptive home.

The negative side of the shortage of babies is many adoptive couples who try to adopt privately in an attempt to speed up the process. This leaves pregnant teenagers in a vulnerable position, as some private adoption brokers are paid by adoptive parents and present attractive packages to pregnant young women if they place their babies for adoption. Beware of advertisements offering benefits to pregnant, distressed women, as they may be shady operations that exert pressure to place your baby for adoption without offering support for any other options.

You will find varying degrees of input into the selection of the adoptive parents, depending on the options in your district. You will need to find out your options regarding the degrees of openness versus confidentiality in the adoption process, as they vary from place to place. The options in adoption are mentioned in the section on social workers and are detailed further in my book, *Saying Goodbye to a Baby: A Book About Birthparent Loss and Grief in Adoption* (Child Welfare League of America, 1989).

If you choose adoption, it is important not to be a passive participant in the process. You are the parent until the adoption papers are signed. This means that you have the rights of any other parent to take pictures, dress, feed, hold, and name your baby. You can choose the degree of contact you want with your baby, and no one has the right to keep your baby from you if you desire contact. This is your personal choice. Collecting mementos of the pregnancy, birth, and baby are important, as you will cherish them more and more as time goes by.

Many years ago, I clipped an Ann Landers column from the newspaper. I have kept it because it has seemed to me that I was that "mother of our child." Perhaps you too will feel comforted by these words, should you also choose to give your baby up for adoption:

Dear Ann Landers: I am one of those fortunate women who became a mother through adoption. Hundreds of times I've wanted to say, "thank you, dear girl," to that wonderful young mother who gave up her baby because she knew it would be best for the child. How better to reach her than through Ann Landers? May I?

Dear Mother of Our Child: You have made our lives worth living. You have given us the most precious gift in the world. If you ever wonder if you did the right thing, please know the answer is "yes."
Because of your unselfishness and mature judgment, your little one will get a great deal of love from a mommy and dad and two sets of doting grandparents. And because she is so loved and cherished, she will grow up straight and strong and secure. God bless you. —*Another Mother*

Dear Mother: I am not printing the name of your city. Let thousands of young women believe this letter was for them.

The adoption process takes time, and procedures may vary slightly from place to place. There is often a waiting period of about a week after birth before the adoption process can be initiated. In provincial or state adoptions, social workers are involved in the process. Before final papers are signed, the child welfare social worker makes home visits to the prospective adoptive family over an extended period of time to be assured that the home is suitable. There may also be a waiting period before you sign the adoption consent to allow a period of grace in case you change your mind. Once consents are signed they may be irrevocable. Your social worker should explain all these procedures in detail according to the law in your province or state. You are entitled to your own legal counsel to advise you of your rights and of the procedures. Be sure that you understand any document that you sign because of the lifelong, irrevocable nature of an adoption consent. The details about the process of adoption and adoption options are outlined in my other book, *Saying Goodbye to a Baby.*

Single Parenthood

If you are thinking about keeping your baby, you need to look closely at your reasons for doing it. Being a single mom is a difficult job in itself, but being a young single mom is even harder, as there are increased stresses. At the time your baby is born, you are only just becoming an adult. You probably have not even thought of a career for yourself or a way you might earn decent wages to support yourself and your child.

Being a single parent is becoming more socially acceptable every day. If anything, you may find social pressure from other teenagers to keep your baby and become a single parent. You will need to be a strong person to withstand social pressure and do what is right for you, not what is right for your friends.

In the beginning, it may seem that keeping your baby is emotionally easier for you and may bring many rewards. But down the road it may not be so rosy. What about the times you may want to go out with friends, or go back to school, or marry, and you have the added responsibility of a child? Might you not blame the child for being born because it traps or hinders you?

You may be feeling alone right now and may even have felt alone before you became pregnant. You may be looking to keep your baby because you need to feel loved and to be assured of having someone who will always be there to love you. This baby is "all yours," and so you might feel your baby could fill a gap in your life. But the baby is actually only a helpless infant who needs a lot of love, care, time, and energy from you. The baby will be totally dependent on you to meet his or her needs. And what if your baby becomes ill? In thinking abut whether to keep your baby, you need to think about all of these practical considerations. Ask yourself whether you are meeting your needs or your child's.

Parenting is a difficult task at the best of times. As a single mother, you will find it even harder without the support of a partner. It is difficult to be a parent when you have not had a chance to gain life experiences to aid you, or when you may still be attached to your own parents and may still rely on them. If you do decide to take on this role, ask your social worker about single-parent support groups, day care centers, and groups offering instruction on parenting skills. As single parenting has become more socially acceptable, more support groups to help the single parent have been established.

It can be frightening when the time comes to actually take the infant home in your arms, and no nurses are there to guide you. You are responsible in every way for the baby's well-being. Yours is a serious decision. The baby is not a toy to play with and dress up, but a child who needs food, safety, and shelter, as well as love, to develop into a normal, healthy child. There is a lot to learn, but lots of happy and loving times too.

This responsibility will change your lifestyle greatly. You may need to live on welfare, at least at first, unless you have job prospects and a babysitter right away. Public assistance provides only a bare minimum for essentials. Your budget will be tight, and you will have no funds for extras or entertainment. Some people feel uncomfortable asking for welfare, but you may have no alternative. Limited money can affect other aspects of your life. You might not have enough money to rent the place of your choice. You may not be able to live where you would really like to live. Financial difficulty is only one category of change confronting you, so you should look at the other parts of your life that will be affected as well. Sometimes family members can assist financially to help you keep your baby, so check out all the options for financial support.

Maybe you have family to help you out. Family is your best support system. Your mother or other female relatives may be able to show you how to care for your baby. Some youth remain living with parents or extended family for support. There is a lot of joy in being a mother, and children are a blessing to cherish for a lifetime. Motherhood is a privilege and continually full of wonder and surprises.

Abortion

You may decide to consider terminating your pregnancy by a therapeutic abortion. Abortion has its own built-in time limit, so you must check this option early in your pregnancy because it might take time to arrange for it. You may have difficulty considering abortion for religious or personal reasons. It may seem hard to face, but remember that either giving up your baby for adoption or being a young single mother is also hard to face.

Abortion counseling is available to you. You can learn the details of medical procedures and what to expect emotionally and physically. Your doctor, school counselor, or public health nurse can point you in the direction of abortion counseling resources. Your neighborhood may have youth clinics designed to meet the needs of pregnant teenagers. These free clinics can direct you to abortion counselors and facilities should you feel too embarrassed to go to your family doctor. Planned Parenthood is a great resource with offices all over North America.

Abortions are safe and legal in North America. Abortion is regulated by the same standards that apply to all medical procedures.* Basically there are two types of abortion: surgical abortions and medical abortions.

Most surgical abortions are performed in the first trimester of pregnancy, within the first 12 weeks following your last menstrual period. They may be done in hospitals, doctors' offices, or clinics, but are usually done in clinics with local anesthesia. The actual procedure takes only about 10 minutes, and you do not need to stay overnight. You can most likely resume your normal activities the following day. Abortions after 12 weeks can be more complicated but are still said to be safer than childbirth.

Nonsurgical abortions are also called medical abortions. They involve taking medication that stops your pregnancy from continuing.

---

* The details of abortion procedures are outlined in Chapter 4 under "Termination."

This must be done within the first seven weeks following your last period. The medication is referred to as RU486, or the abortion pill. It is widely used in France, Britain, Sweden, and China and is available in the United States, but it is not yet available in Canada other than in research trials in Vancouver, British Columbia. This may change, however, so check with Planned Parenthood offices in your area. The Planned Parenthood website (www.plannedparenthood.org) is also a reliable source of information.

Beware of crisis pregnancy centers that may be antiabortion, but are listed in the phonebook under Abortion. They may advertise free pregnancy tests, but do not provide complete information about your options, as they have a strong desire to keep women from having abortions.

Abortions are available everywhere in North America with the exception of Prince Edward Island in Canada. In Canada, abortions in hospitals are free with Provincial Health Insurance as long as the hospital is in the province in which you live. Clinics may be free or may have a fee. In the United States, Medicaid will sometimes pay for abortions for teenagers, and some insurance plans will cover all or part of the procedure. Some accept credit cards. Planned Parenthood will help you find this information, and some Planned Parenthood centers also perform abortions.

You may not feel comfortable telling your parents and may worry that you need their consent to have an abortion. First of all, if you can talk with your parents, this is preferable; you may, however, fear their reaction to your pregnancy or the idea of abortion. Some states require parental consent, but an alternate process is available in which you can speak to a judge to determine if you are mature enough to make your own decision about abortion. Planned Parenthood centers can assist you with this.

In Canada, Ontario and British Columbia allow teenagers to sign their own consents for health care. If you are able to understand what you are agreeing to, which is called giving informed consent, then you will not need to talk to your parents if you do not wish to do so. In all Canadian clinics, your parent's consent is not necessary either if the doctor is clear that you understand what you are doing.

Before having an abortion, you may have to sign a consent that ensures that you have been fully informed about the procedure and the risks. This is also an opportunity to get all your questions answered. You will also acknowledge in the consent that you have been counseled on all the alternatives to abortion and that you have chosen this option of your own free will.

Abortion may cause sadness, a sense of loss, guilt, ambivalence, or relief. The sense of loss might resemble the feelings one has in other kinds of losses but may vary in relation to how early in the pregnancy the abortion is performed. Abortion may also provide you with great relief, which can counteract the negative feelings.

Abortion is a personal choice. Some people regard it as morally wrong. Others only think of it as a great relief from a very stressful situation. You may have mixed feelings about abortion as an alternative to motherhood. It is best to seek counseling to find out more about the physical and emotional consequences of abortion. Pressure from boyfriends or family either for or against abortion may make this a difficult consideration. Remember, it is you who are deciding, and it is you who ultimately has to live with the decision, not anyone else.

Decisions

Whatever you decide, it is just the beginning. Acting on your decision is the hardest part. All of these choices have their drawbacks, and you must select what is best for you. We are all different and have varying resources, strengths, and weaknesses. It is time to look at your needs and those of the child-to-be and understand why you are choosing one course over another. You will need to weigh your emotional side against your intellectual side as you make the decision.

Your decision is likely to be the most difficult you have had to make so far in your life, as it affects another human being. Most importantly, you must be sure that it is your own decision and not one you have made to please others. You don't want to regret it later, nor blame others for their influence. The clearer your thinking is as to your self-determination, the easier it will be to live with your decision afterward. You will know that it was *your* decision, and you will know the reasoning that led you to it. You will be sure that it was the best decision you could have made at the time that you made it. It is always easier in hindsight to look back and say "what if?" or "if only." We are all good at that. But at any given time in your life, all you can do is weigh the pros and cons and then make your decision and learn to live with it.

Yours is a major decision affecting not only your own life but the lives of others and the life of your unborn child. Because of the gravity of the consequences, your physician will probably refer you to a social worker through the local child welfare agency, or you may choose to refer yourself beforehand. It is often helpful to discuss this type of decision with an outside party who is removed from the emotional elements and has no vested interest in pushing you in one direction or another. Your social worker will try to help you make your own decision.

Once you have arrived at a decision, whatever that decision may be, your ability to put your life in order and give direction to your plans for the coming months will be greatly improved. Once your decision is made, find out as much as you can about what it entails to prepare yourself as much as possible for the consequences. Clarifying the unknown helps a great deal to prevent your being taken unaware. If you decide to continue with the pregnancy, it is important to realize that no decision will be final until after you give birth. You will not truly be able to know what to expect until then because giving birth and seeing your baby is an amazingly powerful physical and emotional experience that can overturn any preplanned decision.

Changes Ahead

Pregnancy is not an isolated event in your life. You will find that this change will have a ripple effect on other aspects of your live. Similarly, your present circumstances will affect your decisions. A reciprocal, circular process is occurring. You are being affected by your environment, yet you have the power to act on your environment, to influence environmental conditions through your own actions.

The diagram on the next page is a model of you in the context of your total environment. Various areas of your life overlap and interconnect. This diagram illustrates the potential stresses and the potential

You and the Systems in Your Life

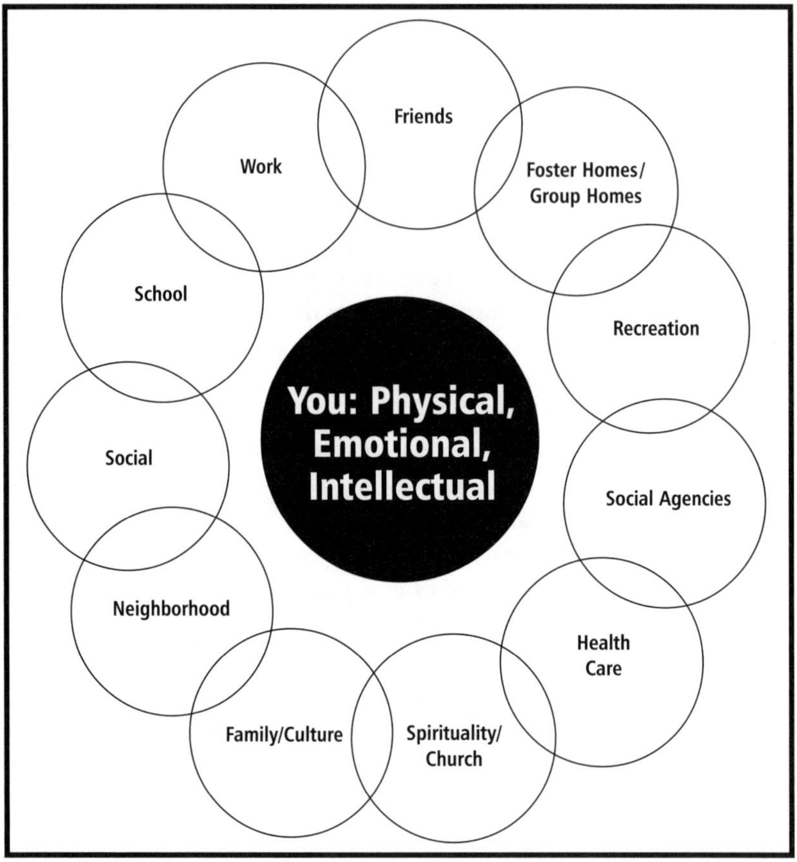

Friends

Work

Foster Homes/
Group Homes

School

Recreation

You: Physical,
Emotional,
Intellectual

Social

Social Agencies

Neighborhood

Health
Care

Family/Culture

Spirituality/
Church

supports in your life. This larger perspective is important to keep in mind as you make decisions about your pregnancy. In making decisions about your pregnancy, you are simultaneously making decisions about other segments of your life.

Look at the diagram above and identify the systems having the most important influence on your life. Count the number of people with whom you can talk and to whom you can turn for help. There may be people whom you have not thought of who are in a position to offer you support. You may feel that you can handle this all on your own, as

I did at first. But your thoughts, feelings, and fears can multiply to the point where you may feel as though you will burst. It is not easy to seek help, but it can be frightening and isolating trying to tackle everything alone. To have someone to confide in and lean on can be a great comfort and relief.

During adolescence, you are already facing numerous changes as you increase your independence, become comfortable with your sexuality, establish your personal identity, and plan for your vocation. Finding yourself pregnant during adolescence compounds the complex issues that you are already struggling with and adds further issues because you are thrust into making adult decisions before you feel ready. As a teenager, it is confusing to be treated as a child sometimes and as an adult at other times. Pregnancy is associated with the adult role and thus will add to further role confusion.

There will be changes ahead in many parts of your life. These changes will vary depending on the decisions you make. Changes require adaptation; adaptation requires flexibility. The more flexible and less rigid you are, the more easily you will adapt to these changes. Remember that all the circles in the diagram represent not only people around you who are affected by your pregnancy, but also possible resources to draw on for help in coping with the changes.

Chapter 2

Looking After Yourself

Two types of resources are available to you to help you with your problems: your own internal resources and the external resources in your environment. Your own inner resources play a major part in how well you will cope with this crisis. Your perception of yourself is crucial. A strong sense of your own worth along with strong self-determination are two of the basic ingredients that will pull you through this difficult time.

Your self-concept includes your self-worth, your self-esteem, and your self-confidence. You must not neglect your self-concept. In fact, this is a time to nurture yourself. You need to strengthen your positive feelings about yourself. You will need to remind yourself of your good points, and we all have good points. Remember that you are still the same person you have always been. You will need to value yourself, like yourself, and accept yourself, if you expect others to value, like, and accept you. Self-respect must come before others will respect you. Be good to yourself. Don't put yourself down. We all make mistakes, and we all have problems at one time or another. No one is perfect. Avoid burdening yourself with excessive self-reproach and avoid blaming others. Guilt and blame are futile and destructive and only lead to lowered self-esteem and self-punishment.

It is easy to doubt yourself and put yourself down right now. The lower your opinion of yourself, the more vulnerable you will be to remarks or criticism from others. If you value yourself and have some self-confidence, the remarks or questions from others will bounce off more easily, and you will not be devastated by them. The lower your self-confidence is, the more you will tend to take the remarks of others personally.

Try to think positively and have faith in your abilities. Believe it or not, you will get through this experience. Your self-concept may become bruised, but it will heal if your self-determination remains strong enough to build yourself up again. Even though you will never forget this experience, it will become a part of your past. It will always remain a sensitive area for you, but the better you deal with the issues now, the easier it will be to put it behind you as a growth-enhancing experience. If your pregnancy becomes a subject you fear ever talking about again, you may create a block to your future growth.

Hindsight is wonderful. It is always easy to look back and wish you had acted differently. But you can't change the past. What you can do is shape your present and your future.

Your pregnancy will set you to thinking about your priorities. You will begin to evaluate what is important to you and who is important to you. You may realize who your real friends are and whom you can trust and rely on. This is a time to take control of your life and your future rather than letting events control you. This is a time to set short-range and long-range goals for yourself. If you have a goal to work toward, it can help you maintain your self-determination. Goals provide you with a positive purpose to channel your energy into.

Don't let this crisis hold you back from your dreams. Your life is not ruined. It may be a setback in some ways, but in other ways you will be maturing, possibly far ahead of your friends. You will experience and learn so much in such a short period of time. No matter how low you feel, the positive aspects of this experience can be built on to rebuild your life. This will be a life-changing event.

External Resources

You can rely on your inner resources to a large extent, but you will also need to rely on external resources. This means accepting help from those around you. Asking for help can be a difficult task in itself, but sometimes everyone needs someone to lean on. No one exists and survives in isolation.

During this time, you will need all the emotional support that you can find. You may feel headstrong and feel the need to prove your independence. That desire to prove yourself to others can also leave you feeling isolated. There will still be times when you will find it comforting to have someone to talk with, someone to share with, someone to just listen to you, or someone to hug. Just having one person who understands what you are going through can make a world of difference.

As a teenager, you may be running scared and fear turning to anyone for help. You may fear that no one will listen to you, and no one will understand you. You may fear that people will judge you or try to persuade you to do something you don't want to do. You need to know that there are people who care about what happens to teenagers. There are people who care about girls who are frightened and confused by their pregnancy. You must not try to hold it all inside and go it alone. Even after everything is over, you may still need to talk with someone about your experience to get it off your chest and out of your system so that you may get on with your life.

Receiving positive feedback from others is another way of preserving your precious self-concept at a time when you may be doubting yourself and your decisions. Or you may need to rely on someone for help with practical matters. Both emotional and practical support may come from family, friends, boyfriends, teachers, social workers, school counselors, nurses, doctors, volunteers, or your religious community.

There are crisis centers to call if you just need someone to talk with in a confidential manner. You can call a crisis line for any reason, and this might be a good place to begin if you are not sure where to go for help. Workers at the crisis center can put you in touch with resources appropriate for your needs.

Chapter 3

Telling Others

Telling others is part of your acceptance of your condition and part of taking action. It is often your fear of telling people, especially parents, that postpones your own decisionmaking. Should you be considering abortion, you may postpone telling those who might be in a position to help you. Postponement often results in having abortions later rather than early in pregnancy. Abortions in late pregnancy are difficult both physically and emotionally.

Letting out your secret will give you tremendous relief. But it is hard to find the right moment or the right words. It will not be easy, so it is helpful to choose the person easiest to tell and tell that person first. This will give you some idea of what the next person's reaction may be and will help you to become comfortable with disclosing the information. Most likely, the first person will be either your boyfriend or your best friend, as during adolescence you are often closer to your peers than to your family. You may find it easier to tell friends because they are your own age and are not as emotionally attached to you as your parents.

Think through your worst fears. What is the very worst reaction you might encounter? Usually we worry about things that never happen, and most likely the reactions of those close to you will not be as terrible as your worst fears have led you to expect. How people react will depend largely on the relationships you have with them. If you have a caring relationship, then the chances are their reactions will come from caring attitudes. If you have had difficulties, for instance, with your family, then naturally this will be a more difficult process for you. Remember to line up as many supports as you can, because if you have a strong negative reaction from one person, then you can find refuge in another.

Plan where, when, and how you will explain your dilemma. Thinking it through and rehearsing it in your mind will make it easier. Set a date and stick to it. Procrastination causes only more worry by delaying the inevitable. It is inevitable that you will tell someone, even if that someone is the health-care professional you tell to find out about abortion. Whom you will tell may well depend on your decision, because if you choose abortion, you might not have to tell family or friends. But if you choose to carry the baby to term, then your condition will become apparent. You will also have to think about relatives other than the immediate family and decide whether you want them to know. If you want them to know, who will tell them?

You may feel uncomfortable and ashamed and wish you could run away and not tell anyone at all. It is possible to move to a group home for pregnant teens out of town, but you will still be faced with the same people when you return. I chose to tell very few people but found that word got around quickly anyway. It would have been much easier for me in the long run to be up-front about the fact that I was pregnant. Keeping a secret requires a great deal of energy, and even more energy is expended in the cover-up. I can only regret that I did not have enough self-confidence and faith in my friends to be open and honest. In retrospect, it is my impression that I would have had a lot more support from my friends than I had imagined. But my fear of rejection did not allow me to rely on their friendship.

Telling others of your pregnancy will be an emotional time for you. You may cry, and others may cry. Remember, each person you tell will go through emotions similar to those you have been going through. Shock and disbelief will come before acceptance and logical thinking.

Boyfriends

Remember that although you feel totally alone, there is a young man somewhere who was equally responsible in the process of conception.

You need someone to share your burden, and he is logically the first person to speak to, as he too is part of this. You may fear he will push you away or blame you, but he may be a source of comfort and strength to you.

His feelings and fears may be similar to yours. Telling him may be a relief. He can be a shoulder to cry on and someone to talk with about what you are going to do. He may have his own ideas about what is best to do, but keep in mind that you must make the decision in a well-thought-out manner and not to please anyone, as you do not want to regret your decision or blame him later.

Your boyfriend may be in shock at first and may feel trapped himself. He may even offer to marry or move in with you because he may believe this is the right and responsible thing to do. Wait until the overwhelming emotion has subsided before trying to discuss the issue, because you'll need to be in a rational frame of mind. You cannot discuss anything when you are upset, even though you may feel it is urgent that you take some decisive course of action.

Your boyfriend is often the one who is left out in the process of your pregnancy. Although you may be overwhelmed by your own needs right now, don't forget that your boyfriend will have needs too. He may benefit from discussing them with someone because he may also need information and support. He may fear that he will be forced to pay money that he doesn't have, or he may fear rejection from his family or your family, who might blame him for your predicament. You should make him aware of the professionals in youth clinics and child welfare agencies who are available to help him.

Friends

When you are a teenager, your friends are a vital part of your life and are associated with your self-worth. As you may be closer to your friends than to your family at this stage in your life, their acceptance and approval is central to your self-esteem. You probably fear the stigma of your condition and fear being ostracized. Actually, teenagers today often pressure girls to keep their babies, as this is becoming a more socially acceptable route. Peer pressure can be well-meaning but can push or pull you in directions that you might not choose for yourself, because the need to belong to the group and to be accepted by it is so strong. You will need to hang on to your self-determination. Some friends may want to advise you, but they are not going through it; *you* are.

Friends may be curious when they notice that you are putting on weight. They may draw their own conclusions, tease you about getting fat, or ask you questions directly. On the whole, friends mean well when they inquire, but all too often there is at least one nosy person in every crowd who has big ears and a sharp tongue. Unfortunately, some people still thrive on other people's problems and relish a good piece of gossip; friends, however, still have the potential to be genuine supports. Just one good friend who cares may be enough to help you through this experience.

When your friends find out about your pregnancy, they may be scared and avoid you. Pregnancy has hit close to home, and it reminds them how vulnerable they are themselves. If you became pregnant, maybe they could too!

Confiding in friends may be very helpful when you are getting back into the swing of things later. If you decide to go through with the pregnancy, you may leave school temporarily or attend an alternate school. Friends can keep you in tune with what is going on and help you get accepted into the system when you return.

Family

Telling your family will probably be the hardest step of all. You may fear disappointing them or letting them down as their daughter. You may fear their rejection or dread their lectures. Once again, be aware that your parents will have to go through their own state of shock and emotions before they can accept the facts and think them through. So, the first reaction you will find will be an emotional one. Emotional reactions are hard to take regardless of whether they are reactions with crying or with shouting. Because of the emotional elements in telling parents, you will probably try to put it off as long as possible. Don't forget that your parents' hugs can be the most comforting.

Parental reactions may be anything from overprotection to rejection. On the overprotective side, they may wish they could go through this themselves instead of you. On the rejecting side, they may kick you out of the house and overreact for reasons of their own. Parents who are upset may say things that they don't really believe. In the heat of the moment, they may call you names. Parents may even blame each other. If you are one of those girls unfortunate enough to have rejecting parents, remind yourself that it is *their* own failure if they cannot be compassionate toward and understanding of their daughter in need of their help. Possibly underneath they see your pregnancy as a reflection of their own inadequacies as parents and feel they are to blame. Or they may be overwhelmed with their own problems and unable to reach out to you, as they are themselves so troubled. Whatever the reason, if you are left to walk the streets, there are group homes and foster homes where you can go, so contact a social agency. Professionals can offer family counseling to help your family cope with these changes. It is to be hoped that your parents' reaction will fall somewhere between the two extremes. You may be able to predict their reaction by looking at the existing relationship between yourself and your family. How have they reacted to other family problems? Just think what a relief it will be once this bridge is crossed.

Your pregnancy will also affect the lives of your parents, and they too may need someone to talk with. They may wonder if it is okay with you to share this with their friends and relatives. Social agencies and professionals can be a help to parents as well.

Your parents, especially your father, may take their anger out on your boyfriend. They may attempt to cut off your relationship, if you are still seeing him, and this may be another hurdle to cross. Parents may blame him, as it is easier for them to see him as solely responsible, rather than their daughter, who is a reflection of themselves. Parents often forget that it takes two to conceive a child, and two people are responsible, not just one. Some parents blame their daughter and have different expectations of young men. People still tend to adhere to the belief that sexual experience for males is okay but for females it is not, so the responsibility for birth control usually rests with the female.

If you have brothers and sisters, they can be good supports. Being closer in age to you, they may understand your feelings more easily, and you may find it easier to talk with them. They may help you gauge your parents' reaction. Just their kindness, acceptance, and company can be comforting, even if you can't talk at length. They may have questions and may want to help but may not know where to begin. Your siblings are likely to feel upset and worried about you. They too may wonder if it is okay to tell their best friends, or they may be apprehensive about anyone at school commenting or asking questions about you.

The more comfortable you are about your pregnancy, the more comfortable your family will be in talking with you or others about it. It will be up to you to provide the direction as to how comfortable you are. The more accepted the fact is at home, the less anxiety there will be surrounding the topic and the more communication there will be. The more secrets there are, the more barriers and tensions there will be concerning "no-no" areas of conversation. You may find your family avoiding the topic of pregnancy because they fear it is too painful for you and that you might get upset. So you must set the tone.

Family crises always seem so terrible at the time, but it is during these crises that we have the potential to enrich our relationships with our families. This crisis may bring your family closer than they have ever been, or it may drive in a wedge to push them further apart. Try to use the occasion of telling your parents as an opportunity to be genuine and open and to bring yourself into a closer relationship with your family.

School

If you choose abortion, your schooling will not be interrupted. If you choose to continue your pregnancy, however, it is likely to disrupt part of your school year. Making a decision about your education is critical right now. Sometimes, girls drop out of school and are later seriously affected by the loss of education. If you decide to abandon school completely, you will be socially disadvantaged in planning for long-term goals. In the short run, it may seem an easy way out and a way to avoid facing others at school.

Some programs for pregnant teenagers offer academic courses as well as prenatal education, day care, and child care instruction. You are more likely to find these alternate programs in larger centers. Tutoring and correspondence courses are available, or your school may send work home for you to complete if you feel embarrassed about returning to your regular classroom. Group homes have teachers available for you so that you can continue your courses. You will need to speak with your school principal about the options available in your area or in other vicinities. You may choose to move to a group home or to another community to participate in a special school program.

So this means telling your school about your pregnancy. If you do not feel comfortable about contacting your school, your parents, a school counselor, or a social worker could do this on your behalf. A professional who works with pregnant teenagers is likely to know about these school programs and may be able to assist you in looking at your opportunities. Just remember that alternative schooling is available.

Your school may base its expectations for your completing the school year on your past record. If you have been a good or average student, the school often looks more favorably on your situation and may take past grades into account. If school has been difficult for you all along, however, you may have to work harder to pass your grade. Any time missed could put you seriously behind and cause you to take longer to catch up.

You may feel that everything is ruined, even your education. This does not have to be the case. There are ways of working it out so that you can save your year, but you must speak up and talk with people who can help you arrange this.

Chapter 4

The Pregnancy

Physical and Emotional Changes

During adolescence, you are already in a time of physical and emotional change. If you decide to carry your baby to term, you will find that pregnancy compounds these changes. Pregnancy brings its own set of physical and emotional alterations. Your body will change physically. Your hormonal balance will change. Your moods will fluctuate.

Because your body is still growing, you require extra nutrients. Pregnancy and growth together put extra demands for nutrients on your system. Your body is still developing at the same time that the fetus is developing. Regular meals including a variety of foods from all the food groups are essential to your own health as well as to your baby's health. Junk food such as French fries, soda pop, and potato chips may satisfy your cravings but will only add pounds without proper nutrition. You'll only have to take off this extra weight afterward. If you feel the urge to munch, pizza is a better choice than many fast foods because it contains nutrients with cheese, meat, and vegetables. Now is not a good time to start dieting. It may harm the baby.

You can expect to gain 20 to 25 pounds during the full nine-month period. It may be hard to resist the urge to overeat. It is common to overeat under stress. Stress may make it twice as difficult for you to maintain self-discipline. You may turn to overeating as a way of comforting yourself. But watch the weight gain, or you will find yourself dealing with an obesity problem later.

The more weight you gain, the more stretch marks you will be left with, as your skin stretches to compensate for the rapid increase in body size. Stretch marks will fade in time. Using moisturizers may help you retain your skin's elasticity, as will exercise, but most likely you will be left with some stretch marks around your breasts, thighs, stomach, and buttocks. No magic cream can prevent stretch marks.

You may feel awkward as your body changes shape. Eventually you will not be able to fit into your favorite blue jeans and will have to look for looser fitting clothes. You will find looser clothes to be more comfortable. You can make or buy fashionable maternity clothes, or you may find that you already have some loose clothing that fits.

There are other physical changes that you may have to deal with:
• Morning sickness—nausea or vomiting upon waking
• Leg cramps
• Dizziness
• Constipation
• Fatigue
• Increase in frequency of urination
• Tenderness in breasts
• Lower back pain (later in the pregnancy)
• Oversensitivity in teeth to hot and cold

Some doctors caution against intercourse during the last weeks of pregnancy.

Take time to read and ask questions about the stages of your pregnancy so that you can be aware of the physiological changes you should expect. The greater your understanding is of what to expect, the easier it will be for you to maintain your health. If you are planning to give your baby up for adoption, you may feel embarrassed about asking questions or may feel it is not legitimate for you to ask, but this is your body. You are going through the pregnancy, and you have just as much right as any other pregnant adult to know all the details.

Your health is very important to you and to your baby. Regular medical checkups are essential. You may feel embarrassed or uncomfortable with the internal examinations, but before you know it, you will get used to them. Alcohol is to be avoided during pregnancy, even in small quantities. Alcohol binges are dangerous. Smoking can contribute to small, premature babies.

Prenatal instruction is a must. You may prefer a prenatal class for teenagers, especially if you are planning to place your baby for adoption. You would likely feel uncomfortable attending a group with adults who are chattering about their babies and other children. Your family doctor or public health nurse will be able to refer you to suitable prenatal classes. If you are in a home for pregnant teenagers, it will probably offer prenatal instruction for its residents. Prenatal classes are usually conducted by a nurse who discusses the birth process and teaches you breathing to assist you during labor. You may have a lot of questions, and this is the proper forum for discovering what to expect during labor and delivery. Knowing what to expect makes you more relaxed and makes labor easier.

The baby's father may come with you to prenatal classes and the delivery if you want. You may also choose to have any other support people, such as your mother or a friend, with you. This is not a time to be alone, and volunteer labor coaches can be arranged.

During your pregnancy, you will need a balanced combination of rest and exercise. You will be able to remain fairly active. In fact, if you keep your muscles toned up, it will help your body get back to its original shape. After the baby is born, you will be very concerned about looking like your old self again.

There will be times when your mood will be elevated. You will feel elated and will have extra energy. At other times, your mood will be lowered, and you will feel depressed and tired. You may find yourself overreacting to situations in an overly sensitive manner. You may cry for no special reason. These are all normal parts of the emotional changes associated with pregnancy.

The more difficult or unstable your social situation is, the more floods of emotion you may expect. You may be anticipating changes ahead that are laden with emotions, such as giving your child up for adoption, becoming a single mom, or moving in with the father. You may have even married by now and may be adapting to new roles. All these changes can take a toll on your spirits and affect your moods.

Not all emotions are negative. You may experience new positive emotions associated with the miracle of the baby growing inside your body. You may be excited as you feel the baby's first movements. You are likely to develop a feeling for and an attachment to this baby growing inside you. It may feel as though the baby is an extension of yourself. Regardless of the outcome of your pregnancy, you will always remember these good feelings. You will not have only negative feelings to recall. You will learn a great deal from the experience of the pregnancy itself, and what you learn will enhance your life experiences as a whole.

Delivery

In preparation for going to the hospital to deliver your baby, you will probably have packed an overnight bag with nightclothes and personal items. You are sure to appreciate these little items during your hospitalization. You will try to plan around your due date, but this may not be the exact date. Babies do not arrive by the clock, and unfortunately, babies often decide to appear in the middle of the night.

When your labor begins, you will feel your abdominal muscles tighten and relax periodically. These contractions of your uterus will gradually increase in frequency and duration. At the beginning, the sensation will feel similar to cramps in your stomach or cramps during your period. You will time the contractions and depart for the hospital when the interval between the contractions is approximately three minutes in length. Your doctor will give you specific instructions about when to arrive at the hospital. When the contractions are very strong and they occur every three minutes, you may feel as though you will give birth to the baby at any minute, but you generally still have plenty of time. Unfortunately, we all hear the horror stories about prolonged, difficult labor. We rarely hear about the short, easy deliveries. Sift through the rumors you have heard, and be selective about what you listen to. These stories only serve to implant fears in your mind, and they may not resemble your labor and delivery. Women's experiences during labor vary. If you focus on the pain, it will feel worse. Try to distract yourself by concentrating on something else.

The amniotic sac may break before or after you arrive at the hospital. This is often referred to as the time when your water breaks. You will know when this happens because a watery liquid will be released through your vagina.

Once in the hospital, you will be placed in a labor room, which is like a private room. You will be allowed to have someone with you. You should make arrangements in advance for a companion to be with you. It will be comforting to have a hand to hold. You might ask a boyfriend, girlfriend, or your mother to stay with you in the labor room. It can be a lonely time and seem endless if you have to go through it alone. The more tense and fearful you are, the more likely your labor is to be prolonged and difficult.

If you are choosing adoption, some people choose to have the adoptive parents at the birth. This can be very emotional, especially as it is hard to know if you will change your decision after the birth. This is your choice.

In the labor room, nurses will prepare you for delivery. They will check you periodically. You may be given an enema to clear out your bowels. They will swab or sponge a disinfecting solution in the genital area. It may seem depersonalizing to have various medical people in and out of your room during this time, but by now you probably won't care about that. You'll just want to get it over with. Pain medication may be given to you periodically and may make you feel groggy.

Once the cervix is dilated and the baby is in position, ready to be born, you may be wheeled into the delivery room. Now, many hospitals have birthing rooms where you stay during labot and delivery as well as after the birth. You may be given a spinal injection, a local anesthetic, or laughing gas to relax you. This will be discussed and decided by your doctor and you beforehand. Once the baby's head is showing, the doctor may have to do an episiotomy. This means that the doctor makes a small cut to allow the baby to come out easily. This incision may require stitches to heal properly.

There is a possibility that your pelvis will be too small for a vaginal delivery or you may have other complications that require a caesarean section. This means surgery to remove the baby. This will leave a small scar on your stomach.

You will see your baby for the first time right after birth, and you may hold the baby at this time. Witnessing the miracle of life is one of life's great joys. Take some time to feel the natural high of this experience and in the life you have created. You worked hard to deliver your baby into the world.

Following delivery, you will be taken to your room to rest. This may be a private room and even the room you gave birth in, or it may be a ward shared with other mothers. If you are choosing to place your baby for adoption, you may feel uncomfortable as you watch others with their babies. You may want to request a private room before your delivery. You will need to prepare yourself for questions from nosy people in your room or on your ward. Someone may ask where your husband is. Their questions may catch you off guard. You will have to decide how you will respond. Remember that you can just say that you do not want to discuss the matter. Try not to be intimidated by the remarks of others. You have no obligation to answer their questions.

Initially, you will feel exhausted and weak. You may feel high or excited. You will be wearing a sanitary pad and will bleed from your vagina for up to several weeks after birth. It is recommended that you use sanitary pads rather than tampons during this time to avoid the possibility of infection.

Your breasts will swell and feel sore. If you are not breastfeeding, then you will receive injections to stop the production of milk. You may be in some discomfort with the stitches and may have to take sitz baths of hot water and Epsom salts. You may feel sore and may need to sit on pillows for a while.

If you are keeping your baby, hospital nurses will teach you about breastfeeding or bottle feeding. Babies are encouraged to breastfeed shortly after delivery, and this can be an amazing bonding experience.

Your stay in the hospital will probably last about one to three days. But if your baby is premature, he or she may have to remain in the hospital a while after you go home. If the baby is born early, his or her body systems may not be fully developed, and he or she may be underweight. Your baby may have to be placed in an incubator to shelter him or her from temperature changes and infection. If your baby is not healthy, a difficult time may be ahead, necessitating tests, diagnosis, and treatment. If your baby is born with an acute or chronic illness, your life could be thrown into further turmoil. Coping with an ill child will compound the issues you are presently dealing with, and the hospital will have a medical social worker to help you.

After the birth of your baby, you may find yourself crying for no apparent reason. You may get "the blues." These are normal and common reactions for all women. You may feel overwhelmed with the reality of whatever is ahead for you. You will still be going through emotional changes along with physiological changes as your body adapts to its new state now that you are no longer pregnant.

During your hospitalization, you will have to register the baby's birth by completing a form. Even if you are placing your baby for adoption, you will need to go through this procedure and give your baby a name. Your social worker will probably go over this form with you.

If you are placing your baby for adoption, you will need to think about the quality of contact you want to have with your baby. It is a misconception that the mother doesn't have to see her baby if she chooses not to. At the very least, you may have to go through the identification process with your social worker. But adoption policies and procedures vary according to the province or state. Some girls imagine that once the birth has taken place, the baby is whisked away as if by magic, and it is all over. This is not true. There are still choices to be made. You may see and hold your baby. Some girls choose to feed and care for their babies. Some people appreciate the time in the hospital with their babies to bond and give nurturing in the first few days of life. Others choose to have little or no physical contact. You may be advised to not see your baby, as others may feel it will be harder for you to place the baby for adoption. Some girls regret it later if they do not take the opportunity to see or hold their baby, and they always wonder what the baby looked like. This is a very personal choice and is something you must decide for yourself.

If you happen to be an adopted child yourself, you may be even more sensitive to these issues because they will evoke feelings about your own adoption. You may find it harder to separate from your baby because of your own feelings. You may find that the less contact you have with your baby, the easier it will be to separate from him emotionally when you leave the hospital. On the other hand, you may feel the need to nurture and love your baby as much as possible in these few days you have together. This is an entirely individual decision that you will make, based on what you know about how you react in other situations. Separations of any kind are usually difficult for most of us, even in the best of times. Relinquishing a baby is a loss, and as in any other loss, you will go through a period of grieving.

When my baby was born, I was completely unaware that I had a choice. I may have reacted differently if I had had time to think about it. Shortly after the delivery, the nurses brought my baby in to me for feeding. I was totally unprepared for this because no one had asked me beforehand if I intended to feed my baby. I felt ashamed and guilty when I said no. I chose not to feed and care for my baby because knowing myself, I was sure that I would have become so attached to her that I would have had a hard time following through on my decision for adoption. I'd have wanted to take the baby home. This would have been an emotional, reactive decision rather than a well-thought-out decision. Getting to know yourself so that you can predict your reaction is all part of the process. It certainly tests your ability to follow through on decisions.

If you have isolated yourself during your pregnancy, you may feel lonely during this time in the hospital. Having your friends visit may make you feel better.

If you are taking your baby home with you, these few days in the hospital will be valuable. You can learn from the nurses about feeding schedules and physical care, such as changing diapers, bathing, and breastfeeding or bottle feeding. You can begin routines to carry on at home. You can learn to feel comfortable holding and caring for your baby. It may be frightening to think that this helpless infant is totally dependent on you in every way, but it will also be exciting to look down at the little child in your arms.

Termination

Some pregnancies result in miscarriages. This is also referred to as a spontaneous abortion. It usually occurs within the first two to three months of pregnancy, usually because there is something wrong with how the fetus is developing.

Termination is another word for abortion. If you choose to end your pregnancy by abortion, you may or may not be aware of the physiological symptoms accompanying pregnancy. Your awareness would depend on how far along you are in your pregnancy at the time of termination.

First-Trimester Abortions (Early Abortions)

Most abortion procedures are done in the first trimester, that is, up to 12 weeks from your last menstrual period. You may choose to have a support person with you during the procedure.

Nonsurgical abortion. You may choose to end your pregnancy in the first seven weeks, which is less than 49 days since your last period, with a nonsurgical abortion. This requires taking pills called Mifeprex or an injection or liquid called Methotrexate. The medicine stops your pregnancy from continuing. You will have to have two or more visits to the clinic to take one dose of medication followed by another dose a couple of days later. You may also be given vaginal suppositories to help expel your pregnancy. You will then experience bleeding and cramping, perhaps heavier than your normal period, that could last from one to two weeks. You would need to go for a follow-up appointment with the clinic a while later. There is a chance that this method might not work, as it is 92% to 95% effective. Prior to taking the medication, you will have to agree to have a surgical abortion if it is not 100% effective. In the United States, this medication is only available from clinics and some doctors; in 2005, it was not yet available in Canada, although this may change.

Therapeutic surgical abortion. Vacuum aspiration or suction curettage is a procedure that involves removing the contents of your uterus by suction or curettage or a combination of both methods. In the clinic or doctor's office, you go into a treatment room where you lie on an examining table with your legs placed into comfortable knee crutches. If you have had a regular gynecological examination, then you will have experienced this position. The doctor places an instrument called a speculum inside your vagina to hold your vagina open so he or she can see the opening of your uterus (your cervix). Local anesthetic is used to numb your cervix so there will be no pain when it is increasingly widened (dilated). Then the doctor puts a small tube into your uterus and uses suction to empty the contents of your uterus, or a metal curette may be used. This procedure is often called a D&C, for dilation and curettage. If you are 10 weeks or more pregnant, the doctor will check the uterus using a curette to ensure no tissue is left behind. The procedure takes 5 to 10 minutes.

Some clinics offer alternatives to local anesthesia if you do not want to be awake during the procedure. They may offer sedation through an IV (intravenous) or nitrous oxide (laughing gas) as a relaxant. Others may offer a general anesthetic that puts you to sleep for a few minutes. You may also be given pain or relaxant medication prior to the procedure. If the abortion is not free, the type of anesthetic will affect the cost of the abortion.

Medication may be used in surgical abortions to decrease the amount of bleeding. Most women experience some cramping during the procedure. You may have some lighter cramping afterward and may need some pain medication to ease this discomfort.

Second-Trimester Abortions (Late Abortions)

Dilation and evacuation (up to 19 weeks). This procedure requires two visits to the clinic or doctor's office. The day before the abortion procedure, the doctor will dilate the cervix as previously described and insert laminaria (seaweed stems) that absorb water to soften the cervix to allow it to dilate more than for the early abortion. You may need some pain medication for cramping after this preparation. The next day, you return, and the procedure is similar to the previous description except that you may receive IV sedation. The doctor removes the laminaria when you are under anesthetic and performs a uterine evacuation using a larger suction and special forceps. The doctor will use a curette to ensure no tissue remains in your uterus. This takes 10 to 20 minutes.

You may receive medication through an IV to help contract your uterus. You are able to walk to the recovery room where you may get sterile IV fluids and be monitored about half an hour. If you had IV sedation, you will need someone to give you a ride home.

Dilatation and extraction (20 to 24 weeks). This procedure is used for later second-trimester abortions and involves two visits to your doctor or clinic. On the first, your cervix will be dilated with laminaria or medication over the course of one to two days, depending on the dilation necessary. Under general anesthesia, once adequate dilation is achieved, all contents are removed from the uterus. The procedure takes 10 to 20 minutes and is followed by an ultrasound to assure that the cavity is empty. You then remain in the recovery room for one to two hours. You would need a ride home because you have received general anaesthetic.

Induction method (20 to 24 weeks). This procedure can only be done in a hospital and requires an overnight stay. It is quite uncommon now. This involves the injection of saline or prostaglandin into the amniotic sac that induces labor (contractions or cramping of the uterus), and the expelling of the fetus.

Second-trimester abortions are safe surgical procedures and have approximately the same rate of complications as normal childbirth. For safety reasons, it is very important that you inform the clinic about your medical history and any drugs, legal or illegal, that you have taken.

Your doctor will let you know what aftercare is necessary and what follow-up care is recommended after the abortion. You may need to return to the clinic or doctor for a check up. They will be concerned about your physical and emotional health. Counseling is available before and after the abortion.

By having an abortion, you may be able to keep the knowledge of your pregnancy fairly quiet and private. You may not tell anyone at all or you may tell only close friends. This may make your life easier in some ways, but it may also result in a feeling of being isolated or lonely afterward. Your experience with the abortion and your values will determine your emotional reaction to the abortion. You may feel sadness, loss, guilt, or relief. Abortion is a loss, and so you may feel yourself go through a grieving process. Feelings are further complicated by sudden hormonal changes that occur when a pregnancy ends.

For the two to three weeks post-abortion, you must not do anything that could introduce bacteria into the uterus. This means that you must not have intercourse, use tampons, douche, take baths, or go swimming. The cervix remains dilated for a while, and bacteria that enter the uterus can cause serious infections or even pelvic inflammatory disease. Symptoms associated with infections are an elevated temperature, heavy or foul-smelling discharge, and abdominal pain.

Remember that it is possible to become pregnant right after your abortion. This is an opportune time to discuss birth control with the clinic counselor or doctor. Abortion is not a healthy birth control method.

Chapter 5

Returning from the Hospital

Whatever decision you make, whether it be abortion, adoption, or keeping your baby, you will eventually be returning from the hospital. The environment you are returning to may be different from what it was before you left. Circumstances may be altered or may appear to you to be different because you have yourself undergone changes. This period of time can be a grey area between endings and beginnings. You may have to face up to people as you put your life in order once again.

Community resource people often believe that the crisis appears to be over and dealt with and may lessen their supportive contact at this time. But this may be a lonely, difficult time as you assume new roles or face new situations. You may be reordering your priorities as you get back on your feet. You may spend time reflecting on what you have experienced and what direction you want to go in from here. Setting goals for yourself can help you to impose order on your life, restore balance, and provide direction.

Back Home to Parents

You may be returning from the hospital after having had an abortion or after having given your baby up for adoption. You may well return to your parents. Your family may react to you just the same as before, as though nothing had happened. But inside you may feel as if a lot has happened. Your parents may still treat you as a child, whereas you may feel as if you have grown up a great deal. You have been thrust into an adult world of decisions and responsibility. You may find it strange that those around you are not aware of these changes in you. Alternatively, your parents may be more restrictive than before. They may not trust you and may worry about your dating for fear of a second unwanted pregnancy.

You may have been living for a while with relatives away from your parents' home. Or you may have been living in a group home or a foster home. Your parents may have even forced you to leave home when they found out that you were pregnant. So you may have begun to develop an increased sense of independence. You have learned to make decisions for yourself and may now be faced with readapting to your parents' lifestyle and rules. This could be an opportune time for discussing and renegotiating their rules. Roles have shifted and everyone has to adapt. Things are not exactly the same as they were before your pregnancy.

If your parents refuse to let you return home, then you will be faced with another new situation. This might mean living in a foster home or a group home. It might mean moving in with a friend or a relative or living on your own. If there is conflict in your parents' home, you may choose to live elsewhere rather than returning to your family.

To live on your own, you will need an income. If you are a minor, it can be difficult to get welfare to support yourself away from home. Welfare authorities usually expect your parents to assume financial responsibility for you. They would be likely to approach your parents, and your parents may tell them that you are free to come home any time. If your family is experiencing problems that make it too stressful for you to return home, child welfare agencies will find some place where you can live. They may place you in a foster home, in a group home, or with a relative, or may arrange for you to collect welfare. A social worker would have to discuss this with your family and obtain their consent. If your parents refuse to give their consent, then the social worker would have to take the matter to court to obtain temporary custody of you. The social worker will take your family problems seriously and will first attempt to help you work out the difficulties with your family. He or she will see placement as a last resort. There are also homes available on a crisis basis for short-term needs.

The Single Parent

Keeping your baby is a courageous decision that brings both the joys and challenges of parenthood. Lots of changes will happen quickly. You may be faced with making it on your own as a single mother. Leaving home can be traumatic for a teenager even under the best conditions. For you, it will be one more change in the midst of many other simultaneous changes.

You may initially decide to return to your parents' home, as this may provide you with a home base, a sense of safety, and a feeling of security. You may need time to find accommodation and sort out finances. There may be too many changes to make at once, so remaining at your parents' home may allow you to make the changes a step at a time.

Whether you decide to stay with your parents, stay with friends or relatives, or live on your own, you will be entitled to financial assistance from welfare. You should apply for welfare as soon as possible. Welfare provides only a mere subsistence level of income for you and your baby, and you may find it hard to find suitable accommodations on this monthly income. You may be able to supplement this amount through part-time employment, although extra earnings over a certain amount may reduce your welfare check.

To provide yourself and your baby with adequate housing, you may have to consider sharing an apartment or applying for public housing. Public housing is subsidized by the government, so there are usually long waiting lists for accommodations. Another alternative is cooperative housing. This is not public housing. It is nonprofit housing operated on a cooperative basis and administered by a board of directors. Often, subsidized units are available for low-income families, but even the regular rental units offer reasonable rents because it is not intended that the buildings be rented for profit. There is usually a social component in these complexes that is an added attraction. Cooperatives offer a sense of ownership, as the building is actually owned by the residents.

Rent pays for the mortgage and upkeep of the building. Each tenant does not actually own his or her suite but has a share in the total ownership by this contribution of rent and has input into decisions about how the building is operated. More information about cooperatives can be found by calling cooperative organizations listed in your telephone directory.

You will also have to budget for items for your baby. You will need a crib, a stroller, and baby clothes. Even if you manage to get some items given to you or are able to purchase them secondhand, the costs can mount up. It could prove helpful to work out a monthly budget to make your money stretch as far as possible.

Some have supportive parents to lean on during this transition while others are not so fortunate. If you do return to your parents' home, there could be a potential for conflict. They will still relate to you as their child. At the same time, you will be establishing your identity as an adult. You may struggle to assert your independence in your new role as a parent. It can be difficult to separate and establish your autonomy while you are still dependent on your parents. If you are living under their roof, then you will still be dependent on them.

Your roles as parent and homemaker may overlap with your mother's roles as parent and homemaker. This is a time to define who does what and, especially, who does what with the baby. You may resent your mother's advice and feel she takes on too much of the mothering role with your baby. Your mother may feel you rely on her too much and may resent being a free live-in babysitter. Sometimes two mothers in one house and one kitchen can be too much. But for financial and emotional reasons, you may decide the positives outweigh the negatives. You may find this is your best option for the time being. Your mother can be a great resource and support.

Having the support of your parents may allow you the opportunity of returning to school or completing a job-training course. Help from your mom may be crucial when you first bring the baby home. You will feel tired and will appreciate the extra help. Your mom can probably provide you with useful tips about caring for your baby.

During this time, you may appreciate support from the baby's father even if you and he no longer maintain a relationship. He may offer to babysit to provide you with some time for yourself. You may have a boyfriend who is not the baby's father, and he may be a great help to you in both practical and emotional areas.

As a single parent, you may find it difficult to get back with your old crowd of friends. Your needs may be different, and you may find yourself drifting toward new friends. If you leave school, you will cut off your major avenue of social contact. You will need to find new opportunities to make friends. Because you are still a teenager, staying in contact with friends is important.

Various social groups and parent-support groups available for single parents can afford you the opportunity to share common problems with other single parents, as can drop-in centers for moms and tots. These allow mothers a break and a chance to socialize while the children are cared for and play with other children. Single moms often participate in maintaining day care centers. Some day care centers are operated on a cooperative basis. They survive on the volunteer time given by parents. Volunteering time in a cooperative center may be a good way to meet new friends.

Public health nurses often visit newborn babies and their mothers. They can advise you about the baby's care, health, and development. These nurses are also aware of any community resources such as day care subsidies or drop-ins to help single mothers. Specialized services may be available in your community to meet the needs of single teenage mothers. Some communities have special programs to assist you in completing high school as well as in learning about child care. Some high schools have specific classes designed for young parents. Books on child care and child development are available in any public library.

You may find it helpful to join a parenting group. Society expects us to "just know" how to be a parent, but no one is prepared for these responsibilities. Sometimes it can be reassuring to find out that other parents are experiencing similar difficulties or have similar concerns.

Marriage or Living Together

Babies benefit from having both parents involved in their care. You can share the joys and learn together. Parenting is a big responsibility and a lot of work so two parents can more easily carry the load. You may be in the process of moving in with your boyfriend or husband when you return home from the hospital with your baby, or you may have moved in together in the months prior to your baby's birth. You may also be leaving your parents' home simultaneously. Most likely you have moved to a new neighborhood and into an apartment that you will now have to furnish. Regardless of the sequence of events, you will be adapting to numerous changes in a relatively short period of time.

It may provide you with a sense of security and comfort to have a man around to lean on and to share with, but he may be going through changes too. He may be unemployed. He may have just graduated and may be deciding on a career. He may have left school prematurely and be looking for a job. He may want to continue his schooling. Your partner may feel inadequate as a husband and father and as the breadwinner of his new family. He may need to lean on you for reassurance and support. A new live-in relationship can be fun and exciting, but it is also a big commitment. Strong, lasting relationships need attention and work to overcome challenges.

Your new family may be starting out with financial constraints. If you have to live on welfare, the money provided is minimal. Your budget will be very tight. There will be no funds for extras, especially as you will have the additional expenses for the new baby. Welfare may be able to help you out with some of these extra expenditures.

You may decide to live with one of your parents' families initially until you are able to establish yourselves financially. This may allow some time for your spouse to find a job or time to find an affordable apartment.

Living with your mother, mother-in-law, or boyfriend's mother can be helpful in many respects, but it can have its drawbacks. Any conflicts may spill over into your relationship with your husband or boyfriend. You may get into conflicts with family members about parenting. You may not be able to "set up house" as you had hoped because it is not your house but theirs. The lack of individual space and lack of privacy with your spouse or boyfriend may come at a time when they are most needed. You will need time with your spouse or boyfriend to sort out your new relationship and your new roles. This level of privacy may not be possible if you are living under someone else's roof.

You will find that your social life will change because you have increased responsibilities with a baby, a home, and a spouse. If you have left school, this can radically change your social contacts. If you desire to complete your schooling, you should check into alternative programs in your community.

With the new baby at home, you may find it difficult to get time for yourself or to get out of the house. First you will have to find a responsible babysitter, and then you will have to find the money to pay the babysitter. You may feel tied down with feeding schedules. To go anywhere you have to bundle up the baby and take a bag full of diapers and bottles. It can make going out seem like a big ordeal, especially if you do not have access to a car and have to rely on public transportation.

If you have a close family, they may be able to help you with babysitting as well as help out in other ways. Time out as a couple and time just for yourself are very important and are often neglected once a baby arrives. You will still need to attend to your own needs and the needs of your relationship with your spouse in spite of the demands of the baby. You may feel guilty and believe you are not being a good mother if you leave your baby with babysitters to do something for yourself. But if you feel these needs and don't respond to them, then you are doing yourself and your baby a disservice in the long run. You will only store those frustrations and possibly take them out on someone close to you, such as your spouse or your baby.

Your spouse will also need time for himself. He may want to spend an evening alone or with his buddies. It is important for him to meet his individual needs just as it is important for you. Many couples make the mistake of giving up or neglecting friendships that existed prior to marriage. Later on they find that they have no friends. The more friendships that both you and your spouse maintain, the more supports each of you have.

So in adapting to this new family lifestyle, you and your spouse will have to make room for your own needs, your needs as a couple, and the needs of your baby. You may feel pushed and pulled in various directions with the demands of these new people in your life.

You will need to put energy into your relationship with your spouse. A good relationship does not "just happen." It comes about through a lot of effort and care to maintain open communication. There will be pressure on your relationship because of the demands of the new baby, so you will need to devote extra care and attention to maintaining a strong relationship if it is going to endure over time.

Your relationship will need to be strong enough to weather many up and down times. It is now, while your relationship is still in its beginning stages, that you will be building the foundation for the years ahead. You will develop habits and patterns of relating to each other as you begin to live your life together. It is important to set the tone of your relationship right from the beginning and consciously develop positive, open lines of communication and interaction. When so many changes are taking place, it is easy to neglect vital areas such as nurturing your relationship with your spouse.

Marriages today often end in divorce. Teen marriages have an even greater potential for failure. Teenagers often face additional pressures on their marriages; the younger people are, the less equipped they are to deal with these pressures. These are hard challenges, but not impossible ones. Make sure you have lots of practical and emotional support to add to your own determination and inner strength.

Chapter 6

Birth Control

Once you are no longer pregnant and the peak of the crisis is over, it is time to ensure that you are protected from another unwanted pregnancy. You may believe that it will never happen again, but it can if you do not use contraception during intercourse. Family planning clinics are a necessary resource for you. Prevention of unwanted pregnancy is the ideal. As you know now, pregnancy can happen to anyone and can happen very easily. It is not worth the risk of going through it all again.

A great deal of misinformation is passed around among young people. A lack of information could lead to a second unwanted pregnancy. For instance, some sperm are secreted before ejaculation and pregnancy can even occur without intercourse if sperm are released near the vagina. You can become pregnant after having intercourse for the first time. In the early teenage years, periods can occur without eggs being released, so you may be deceived into believing that you can't become pregnant and have no need for birth control.

Before deciding on a method of birth control, you should learn how your reproductive system operates. This knowledge is crucial if you are to use birth control effectively. Your local library or bookstore will have books on reproduction and contraception. Many excellent websites also offer information on reproduction, sexuality, and birth control (see Appendix D). Family planning and birth control clinics, Planned

Parenthood, your school nurse, your health department, and your doctor can provide you with pamphlets or booklets, give you comprehensive information, and help you decide what might work best for you. You have many options when it comes to decisions about birth control. It is important to plan ahead and be prepared.

Oral Contraceptives: Birth Control Pills

Combined Pill

The most common birth control pill contains two hormones (estrogen and progesterone) that prevent the monthly release of your egg from your ovaries (ovulation). The pill is 99% effective *if* you take it correctly. The pills must be taken on a daily schedule at about the same time each day. If you forget one pill, you need to take the next one as soon as you remember it, even if it means taking two pills on the same day. You would then need to use an additional birth control method to safeguard against the risk of pregnancy that month. In the first week of taking your first month's cycle of pills, you should also use a second method of birth control to be absolutely safe. Birth control pills come in a container with a three- or four-week supply of pills. Some people do not have a menstrual period with the pill; if you miss two periods in a row, you should check to ensure that you are not pregnant. Birth control pills do not provide any protection against sexually transmitted diseases (STDs). They are available only by prescription from your doctor or a clinic. If you get sick and are put on medication such as antibiotics, check with your pharmacy, as other medicines may interfere with the effectiveness of the pill, requiring a back-up birth control method.

Mini-Pill

Another form of the pill is a progestin-only pill that works by reducing and thickening cervical mucus to prevent sperm from reaching your egg. This is about 98% effective. It also needs to be taken on a daily schedule and does not protect you from STDs. This pill is available by prescription from your doctor or clinic.

Condoms

Male Condom

Condoms are widely used among teenagers because they are readily accessible over the counter at pharmacies and in some restrooms, plus they are relatively inexpensive. Some family planning clinics may give condoms away for free. A condom is a thin rubber sheath, like a deflated balloon, worn by the male over his penis during intercourse. It must be in place before any contact occurs near your vagina because sperm may leak out of the penis prior to ejaculation. The condom must not fit too tightly, or it may break during ejaculation. Some space should be left at the tip of the penis to hold the semen and prevent sperm from getting into your vagina. Condoms are more effective when used along with spermicidal foam. This can be an aid in case the condom should break. Foam is more effective with condoms than cream or gel. For the foam to be effective, you must not douche or bathe for at least eight hours after intercourse, but you can shower.

Spermicidal foam disappears by absorption. You must not use oil-based lubricants such as Vaseline, whipped cream, or cooking oil with condoms because they make holes in condoms in a few seconds. If condoms are used correctly, they can be up to 97% effective, and they do provide protection from STDs. This protection from diseases is a major benefit of condoms. Condoms can be used in addition to other birth control methods to add safety as well as STD protection not available with other methods.

Female Condom

The female condom is similar to a male condom. It is made of a thin sheath material, only larger and with a flexible inner ring. It is inserted similarly to a diaphragm. You squeeze the ring and put it as far as possible into your vagina. The ring then covers the cervix. Its sheath material holds the condom in place. The outer ring lines the vaginal wall and helps cover the lips of the vagina. The penis must stay inside the female condom to be effective. The female condom is not as popular as the male condom because it is more awkward to use. It gives you a choice to take responsibility for yourself if your partner does not want to use a condom or does not have a condom with him. It lessens transmission of STDs but does not offer full protection, as there is still more skin-to-skin contact than with a male condom.

Other Contraceptives

Patch

A skin patch is available that is worn on your lower abdomen, buttocks, or upper body. It releases the same two hormones as the combined birth control pill into your bloodstream. It is 99% effective, but appears to be less effective in women who weigh more than 198 pounds. You wear the patch for three weeks and then remove it for one week, which allows for your period to occur. Then you put another patch on. The patch does not protect you from STDs. It is available only by prescription.

Vaginal Contraceptive Ring

This is a flexible ring about two inches across that is placed into your vagina. It releases the same two hormones as the combined birth control pill and is about 98% effective. You insert this ring yourself, and it remains in your vagina for three weeks. You then remove it for one week to allow your period to occur. If the ring comes out of your vagina and remains out for more than three hours, you need to use an additional method of birth control for the rest of the month. There is no protection from STDs. The ring is available only by prescription.

Morning-After Pill

This birth control method is for emergency situations such as unprotected intercourse, two or more days of missed pills, or birth control failure such as a broken condom. You take two large doses of hormones similar to those in the combined birth control pill. The first dose must be taken within 72 hours of intercourse, and the second dose is taken 12 hours later. It reduces the chance of getting pregnant by stopping the release of your egg if given before ovulation occurs. If you have ovulated, it can stop the egg from travelling down and implanting in your uterus. It is 98% to 99% effective. If you are already pregnant, the morning-after pill will not work. It does not cause a miscarriage. A doctor's prescription is not necessary for the morning-after pill and it is available at most pharmacies.

Injection (Depo-Provera)

This injectable hormone (progestin) is given once every three months. It prevents sperm from reaching your eggs and prevents a fertilized egg from implanting in your uterus. It is 99% effective. It does not protect you from STDs. Depo-Provera is only available by prescription.

Injection (Lunelle)

This injection is given once a month and contains the same two hormones as in the combined pill. It is 99% effective, but offers no protection from STDs. It is available only by prescription.

Diaphragm with Spermicide

This is a rubber dome with a flexible springy rim that covers the cervix and acts as a barrier to kill sperm before they reach the uterus. Spermicide gel or cream must be applied to the diaphragm before you insert it into your vagina. It must be inserted before intercourse and stay in place for at least six to eight hours after. It can be left in place for up to 24 hours, and needs to be washed with soap and water before the next use. If you have intercourse again within 24 hours while the diaphragm remains in, you need to add fresh spermicide with a plastic applicator. You need to get a diaphragm from a doctor or clinic where it will be fitted properly for size. If you have a diaphragm that you had been using before a pregnancy, you need to have it checked again, because you may need a different size after a pregnancy, abortion, or miscarriage. If you gain or lose about 20 pounds you may also need a different size. A diaphragm is about 83% effective and needs to be used even when you have your period. It provides no protection against STDs.

Cervical Cap with Spermicide

This is a soft rubber cup with a round rim that fits tightly around the cervix. Like the diaphragm, it must be used with spermicide. It may be difficult to insert and can remain in place for 48 hours without having to reapply spermicide for repeated intercourse. It is necessary to be fitted for a cap by a doctor or at a clinic. It is 83% effective, and has no protection against STDs.

Sponge with Spermicide

This is a small sponge shaped like a doughnut that is coated in spermicide. It is effective for 24 hours. It is about 90% effective and provides no protection against STDs.

Spermicide Alone

Spermicidal creams and foams can be purchased over the counter in any pharmacy. Read the instructions carefully, as spermicide needs to inserted into your vagina before intercourse and remain in your vagina without being washed out for some hours afterward. Spermicides are ineffective methods of birth control when used alone and are designed for use with another barrier method such as a condom, diaphragm, or intrauterine device. They provide no protection against STDs.

Intrauterine Device (IUD)

This is a small, t-shaped plastic device that often has copper on it. A doctor implants it into your uterus. Most brands have strings that hang through your cervix that the doctor uses to remove the device. Some IUDs contain hormones that are released. They can remain in place for many years depending on the type used. IUDs work by preventing sperm and eggs from meeting and preventing eggs from implanting in the uterus. They are 97% effective and provide no protection against STDs.

Abstinence

Abstinence means choosing not to have intercourse at all. When a male ejaculates, the fluid is full of sperm, and if the fluid gets near the opening to your vagina, even if the penis is not in the vagina, it is possible to get pregnant. Sperm are very effective swimmers. A sperm-filled fluid is also secreted long before ejaculation, so if the penis rubs against your vagina prior to ejaculation, sperm can enter your vagina and lead to pregnancy.

Abstinence is the ultimate form of protection from pregnancy as it 100% effective, but it is all or nothing, because there is no halfway method. You must be aware of the risks if you are engaging in sexual contact without intercourse, as emotions can run high, and you can feel pressure to go all the way to intercourse. Some people think they can handle setting limits on sexual activity, and then find themselves in a situation of having unprotected intercourse. You might feel that planning to have sex is calculating and less romantic, but planning birth control methods in case of unplanned sexual activity is the mature, responsible, and safe choice. You cannot depend on your partner to make safe choices for you.

Birth Control—What Doesn't Work

Withdrawal

Some people confuse abstinence with a technique called withdrawal. In withdrawal, the male pulls out his penis before ejaculation. This does not work at all because of the sperm that are present in fluid that comes out of the penis way before ejaculation. It is also hard for men to stop intercourse just before an orgasm.

Rhythm Method

The rhythm method is based on the idea that you have a time when you are most likely to get pregnant around the middle of your cycle and some days that are safer, when you are less likely to get pregnant. This is a dangerous practice if you do not want to get pregnant. Many women, especially young women, have irregular periods, which means that you can never be sure when your ovaries are releasing an egg. Ovulation, that is, the release of the egg from the ovaries, has nothing to do with when you had your last period. It depends on when you will have your next period, and this means predicting the future, which is risky. Basically, there are no days in the month when you are safe from pregnancy. Also, sperm can survive in inside your vagina and uterus for five to seven days. It is also possible to get pregnant during your period, so it is important to use birth control if you have intercourse during your period. You can get pregnant the first time you have intercourse, and you can get pregnant having intercourse in any position. Whether you have an orgasm during intercourse has no relationship with getting pregnant.

Rinsing Sperm Away

Sperm cannot be rinsed away after sexual intercourse by douching (using a device to squirt liquid into your vagina). It is untrue that soda such as cola kills sperm in your vagina. Taking a bath or urinating does not kill sperm. Deodorant vaginal suppositories or vaginal sprays do not kill sperm.

Condom Substitutes

No effective substitutes for proper condoms exist. Some people think that plastic sandwich wrap or plastic bags will work, but they are not made of the same material and can break or slip off.

Safer Sex

Safer sex means not only using birth control methods that work to prevent pregnancy, but also paying attention to the prevention of STDs. STDs, once called venereal diseases, are serious infectious diseases that are transmitted through sexual contact. Some of these infections can be life threatening. Condoms provide one way of decreasing your risk of STDs, and you can add condoms to any other birth control method. Take time to educate yourself about STDs and how to stay healthy, because they can be prevented.

Chapter 7

Social Supports

Social Workers

In dealing with your pregnancy and its aftermath, your first lines of support will be your family and friends. Social agencies are designed to meet the social needs that your family network does not meet. A social agency may provide income assistance, day care, child welfare, education, employment, counseling, and housing. Various social agencies in your community employ social workers and other professionals such as psychologists, youth workers, and child care workers. Their roles differ and are determined by the scope of the agency's responsibility.

The two main agencies you are likely to encounter in the coming months are welfare and child welfare agencies. If you need financial assistance, you will likely come into contact with welfare workers. If you have been employed, you may be entitled to unemployment insurance. If you have been attending school, welfare will likely be your only option. Welfare is often referred to as public or social assistance.

To apply for welfare, you would most likely be required to go to your local department of social services to complete an application form. You may be interviewed at the time about your financial situation. Many welfare offices are busy, so you may have to wait for a worker to see you. This first interview may be followed by a home visit by another worker. At this time, the worker may ask to see documents to verify your expenses, such as rent receipts, or he or she may ask to see your bank statement. Having these items on hand can make this visit progress more smoothly. If you are in immediate need of funds, agency offices can usually process a check for you the same day, or they may issue you a food voucher. Welfare agencies usually offer other services as well as income assistance. They may cover medical and dental expenses, offer personal and family counseling, and help with budgeting. Welfare workers are generally familiar with a range of community services designed to assist people with low incomes. For instance, they may be able to help you obtain furniture or items for your baby. Because you may not be aware of available services, you must tell your worker what you need, or he or she may not explain what services are available.

Child welfare and adoption agencies may be resources for you. If you are feeling pressure from those around you to place your baby for adoption or fear that those agencies might try to take your baby from you, you may hesitate to seek support from them. Child welfare agencies will be concerned with your well-being as well as with your baby's well-being.

Unfortunately, you may have a negative experience with a social worker who is supposed to assist you in making the decision that is right for you. Some social workers let their own ideas of what is best for you and your baby interfere with counseling you about all of the choices open to you. Various agencies tend to counsel "to" a specific solution and promote a choice based on their own bias. This is something to be aware of when approaching agencies, but a range of agencies are available to you, as are a range of workers in these agencies. Unfortunately, as services are fragmented, gaps exist in counseling services for teenagers who need to be informed of all the options available to them, so you may have to search for information about various options by calling different agencies.

If you are considering adoption, you will need to speak with someone at an agency to find out what it entails. You need to know what to expect to arrive at a decision or prepare for the steps ahead. In Canada, many adoptions are handled by provincewide agencies set up for adoption and other child welfare concerns, including child abuse. These agencies may be operated by provincial governments or by Children's Aid Societies, which operate under provincial mandates. They may offer individual, family, or group counseling. They may operate group homes and foster homes. Employees of these agencies might include social workers, youth workers, and child care workers.

In the United States, state care agencies and private adoption agencies have a similar function. In agency adoptions, the agency is responsible for arranging the placement of your baby. The agency assumes guardianship during this interim period, screens and selects suitable adoptive parents, and looks after the legal process just as Canadian agencies do. To be assured of a reliable adoption agency in the United States, you can contact the National Adoption Information Clearinghouse at 703/352-3488.

Private, or independent, adoptions do still occur in both the United States and Canada, although it seems to be a less common practice in Canada. Private adoptions require the services of a third party who arranges the adoption. This third party is often a physician, a lawyer, or a clergyman. This process allows you to have some say about the people who adopt your child. You may even have direct knowledge of, or contact with, the adopting parents. In this process, you do not immediately relinquish your right to an agency, and you may request that your child be returned to you up until the time of the court hearing. As no government regulations oversee private or independent adoptions, you need to be very cautious about what you are agreeing to. Be sure you have a professional social worker or lawyer looking after your needs who is not working for the adoptive parents.

The trend in adoption is that fewer healthy, white babies are available for adoption than in past years. Increased use of contraception, liberalization of abortion practices, and increased numbers of unwed mothers keeping their babies have influenced this trend. This has a positive side of allowing adoption workers to be more selective in choosing adoptive parents. Along with this decrease in the number of babies available for adoption and the high demand for newborn infants to adopt, however, agencies may reject applications for adoption. Even if an application is accepted, there are long waiting lists. This has led to an increase in the number of babies bought and sold on the black market. This process is illegal. Baby brokers stand to make a great deal of money in this illegal baby market. Females seeking abortions may be asked to carry the baby to term and relinquish the baby to a couple in return for money. You need to be aware of this illegal process in case you should be approached in this manner.

Child welfare agencies may also offer such services as day care to allow you to work, or temporary foster care. Foster care for your baby is something you may consider if you need time while you get yourself on your feet. It could provide you with the opportunity to complete a term at school, find a job, or select a place to live. You would still be able to maintain contact with your baby, and yet have the time and energy to set your life in order. It is possible to place your baby for adoption even after keeping him or her for a while, but it may be best for the baby and easier on you if you place the baby from birth.

You may find a wide range of social workers and other helping professionals in a variety of settings. You may find social workers, counselors, psychologists, and nurses at your school. Family service agencies usually employ social workers and psychologists who may offer individual, family, or group counseling; they may offer group counseling specifically for teens. Family service agencies are available to you to help with various types of problems, and they are not committed to a particular choice. Employment agencies may employ various types of counselors and may have counselors for special-need groups such as teenagers. Your community may have women's organizations or women's resource centers whose workers may have varied backgrounds. Some public housing projects employ social workers to assist with housing problems or other social problems. Neighborhood houses or youth programs may offer special programs for pregnant teenagers or teenage mothers. Hospitals and clinics may employ social workers and other professionals capable of providing this assistance. Keep looking until you find someone who can help you get the resources you need. If you live in a rural area these services may be less accessible. You may have to travel to a larger center to find the services you need.

Group Homes

Group homes are small social agencies or are part of larger social agencies. They can be nonprofit private agencies operated by a board of directors, or they can be government agencies. Some homes may be operated by religious organizations, and the extent of the religious component will vary depending on the home.

Group homes usually employ live-in house parents or staff on a 24-hour basis. They may also employ a social worker or youth worker who would be available to you individually as well as in the discussion groups they might lead.

The group home may be specifically designed for pregnant teenagers, or it may be designed for teenagers with a variety of problems. Group homes may give your daily life a structure that you may find helpful in setting your life in order. Some group homes provide too much structure, but you will find that no group home is exactly like another. Look at several homes if you don't like the first one.

Group homes offer peer support and the opportunity to talk about your pregnancy. Just being around other girls who are facing similar problems can be helpful. You will find out that others are in the same boat as you.

Group homes usually have recreational programs or outings, and prenatal classes. The home may give you the opportunity to find some space of your own and some time to yourself, away from the pressures of family or friends. Choosing to live in a group home doesn't necessarily imply that your family is not supportive. You may need some distance from those around you to clarify your thoughts and establish some autonomy. You may even desire to get away from your neighborhood, as you may feel embarrassed about facing people you know. You may choose to enter a group home to complete your schooling or to help prepare yourself for what is ahead.

Group homes vary in their design. Some homes for pregnant teenagers cater to those girls who plan to relinquish their babies for adoption. Some homes may have a bias in favor of this course of action, and that bias may dissuade you from using such facilities. Other homes are more flexible and are open to teenagers with a variety of problems or are open to pregnant teens regardless of the teen's decision. Even if you are choosing to keep your baby, a group home can be a valuable support to you. Some homes are geared toward helping you arrive at a decision about your pregnancy rather than pushing you in any one direction. If you are considering going to live in a group home for an interim period, you should visit the home and ask pertinent questions to select the home most suitable for you. The group home you choose may charge for your residence. The charges assessed may depend on what your parents' income is or it may be paid through welfare.

At a group home for pregnant teenagers, you will meet girls your own age facing similar problems. The girls will come from all walks of life. You will have the opportunity to learn a great deal from their experiences, and you may meet some girls less fortunate than yourself. Your pregnancy will not be a closed topic of conversation at the home. This openness will allow you to talk about your condition, ask questions, and share your fears with others. As a pregnant teenager, you may not find anyone among your friends who has been through the experience, whereas in a group home, you will make friends with other girls who are going through teenage pregnancies. You will not likely find this opportunity elsewhere, except possibly in group counseling sessions for pregnant teenagers at an agency or clinic.

Hospitals and Clinics

Your community may have various hospitals and clinics designed to address both physical and emotional health-related problems. You will find that within this range of health resources, youth clinics, mental health clinics, birth control clinics, abortion clinics, and women's health organizations are designed to meet the specific needs of teenagers. Your local hospitals may offer counseling programs for adolescents, as well as programs for specific physical or emotional problems. Abortion clinics and birth control clinics may be housed under the same roof.

Hospitals and clinics often have multidisciplinary staff who work as a team. A variety of professionals may constitute a team, and that team might be available to you. Team members may be physicians, psychologists, nurses, occupational therapists, social workers, physiotherapists, dietitians, and volunteers. You may at first be unaware of these other team members in medical facilities. They may be valuable resources for you. You may ask your doctor or nurse to meet with them, or your doctor or nurse may refer you to another team member if he or she is aware of your needs.

Because you are pregnant, it is inevitable that you will sooner or later be in contact with either a hospital or a clinic. In a large facility, you may find impersonal service. You may find that everyone is too busy to answer your questions. As a patient in a hospital, you will receive the services of numerous staff members. You may be confused about their roles. If medical complications arise for you or for your baby, there may be even more staff in and out of your room. Try not to be intimidated by this process, and remember that these staff members are there for your benefit. Take time to ask questions about their functions, what they are doing, and why. Often, staff who work in a medical facility are so familiar with their own roles that they assume that you know why they are there.

As a pregnant teenager, you may feel embarrassed and judged by the staff. Part of your feelings may stem from your own sense of insecurity. If you are alone during your hospitalization or clinic visit, you may feel more vulnerable. Unfortunately, some of these judgmental feelings may be very real. You may encounter individuals in medical facilities who maintain a punitive attitude toward pregnant teenagers. Some people still feel that teenagers must pay for their mistakes, and these people are not likely to be warm and supportive. Some hospitals and clinics attempt to screen staff who work with teenagers or who work in sensitive areas such as abortion clinics, but others make no attempt to do so.

If you should come in contact with these negative attitudes, try to maintain your sense of dignity and recognize that these people's attitudes are only a reflection of their lack of sensitivity and warmth as human beings. Their insensitivity is their problem and not yours. You are entitled to receive the same quality of service in a medical facility as the adult or married pregnant woman in the bed beside you. If you have complaints about a staff member's attitude, you can speak with your doctor, the head nurse, an administrator, or the hospital social worker about the difficulty.

Hospitals may become a large part of your life if you should happen to give birth to handicapped or ill baby or if your baby should become ill after birth. Your relationship with your doctor and other health professionals becomes more important. Your baby may have to have numerous specialists in to examine him or her, and doctors may order various tests. Your baby may be in and out of hospitals, or you may be back and forth for clinic visits. You may find yourself frustrated if your doctors do not have all the answers readily available or if the prognosis for your baby's illness is unclear. Transportation back and forth for medical services could be troublesome and costly. Having an ill child can bring about many changes in your life. Caring for a healthy baby is difficult enough.

If your baby is handicapped or has a chronic illness, you may have ongoing medical expenses. If you are on welfare, this may cover some additional costs. If you have added expenses, charitable organizations may be able to assist you. Check with a welfare social worker or a hospital social worker to find out about financial assistance for medical-related expenses.

Giving birth to a handicapped or ill child is something that no one likes to think about, but it can happen and can cause you to feel guilt, sadness, and anger. You may even blame yourself or believe that you are being punished. This possibility emphasizes the importance of talking with your doctor about your baby's health problems. Blame and guilt will only make you feel worse and will not help your baby improve. Remember that staff members such as the hospital social worker are there to help you deal with the emotional as well as the physical components of illness.

Epilogue

As I look back over the course of my pregnancy, a few instances stand out in my memory. One of the most difficult tasks I had to face was telling my parents. I felt as if I had disappointed them and that hurt me. I always thought that they had looked on me as their daughter who could do no wrong. I felt as if I had spoiled their image of me, but more important, I had damaged my own self-image. I had to work hard at rebuilding my self-confidence. For some time, I worried about what others would think of me. I wondered if my peers would reject me and if guys would still want to date me.

My family was very supportive. If anything, they leaned toward the overprotective side. I lived in a small town on the edge of Toronto. I tried to avoid friends and neighbors, but to hide away was impossible. My family doctor suggested a group home for unwed mothers in Toronto. This idea had not occurred to me. I had not thought ahead about how I would cope with the duration of the pregnancy, as it still seemed unreal. I didn't know anything about group homes.

I applied to live in a group home operated by the Anglican church. The home had a waiting period of about a month before I could move in. It seemed scary, as I had never lived away from home. Part of me wanted to get away to where I didn't have to hide from facing people's questions and didn't have to pretend everything was normal.

At the group home, I became comfortable with my pregnancy. I was able to share my experience with other girls and learn about their situations. I made close friends and had to take increased responsibility for myself. The home provided me with space to think and to relax. Yet it was lonely at times, as it was a long way for people to come to visit me.

My boyfriend and his family were supportive from the beginning. My boyfriend tried to do everything he could to help me. Often I was headstrong and refused his help, feeling that I had to get through this on my own.

The loneliest time was during labor and delivery. The doctor and hospital were unfamiliar to me. The group home staff took me to the hospital by cab and left me once we were inside. From then on, I was on my own. I didn't know quite what to expect in spite of the fact that I had attended prenatal classes. It had not occurred to me to ask anyone to accompany me. I didn't know that I could have had someone with me, and I didn't think I'd need anyone. My family was not told that they could be with me. Once again, part of me felt that I brought this on myself, and I would have to face it by myself.

The nursing staff were not particularly friendly or helpful. They did not take time to explain what was going to happen over the next few hours. I was too intimidated and shy to ask many questions, and once the pain medication was administered, it dimmed my level of awareness. I lost track of time. The process seemed endless. After about seven hours at the hospital, I gave birth to a baby girl.

The group home must have notified my family, and my brother phoned my boyfriend. My boyfriend called and wanted to visit right away. I didn't want him to visit as I feared it would be far too emotional for me. I failed to recognize that he had feelings too. He wanted to visit me and wanted to see his baby. His visit was comforting. Our relationship was nearing an end after about a year and a half, regardless of the fact that my parents had forbidden me to see him. The stress of my pregnancy took its toll on both of us and our relationship. This was yet another change for me, as he had been a major support to me during my pregnancy. He had even been to visit my social worker a few times and I found this helpful. This support was virtually gone when he returned home. Luckily, I had a few extremely good friends who helped me feel worthwhile again.

The five days I spent in the hospital were very emotional. I visited the nursery to see my baby. My parents visited once, and my mother saw my baby. The social worker visited, and I signed papers. I registered the birth and named my baby. I went with the social worker to officially identify my baby.

Coming home from the hospital and leaving my baby behind was one of the hardest times I can ever remember. I shall never forget the feelings of sadness and loss. It was like leaving part of myself behind.

I met with the social worker on a couple of occasions after returning home. I had to sign more adoption papers. The social worker told me about the adopting family. Part of me was not sure if I could handle hearing this background information. Another part of me wanted to know more, yet I was afraid to ask many questions. The social worker gave me a couple of pictures of my baby that I shall always cherish.

One of the common questions I am asked is if I ever think about my child. The obvious answer is yes. I always wondered about her and hoped that she was healthy and happy. I always felt sad inside when I thought of her. These feelings stayed inside. You think of it less often and the details of the experience fade over time, yet when you do think about it, it seems as if it all happened only yesterday. As I got older, interest in the details and my child actually increased.

In 1993, I went through an adoption reunion and met my daughter, who was then 23 with two children of her own. This was an incredibly emotional experience, with intense joy and intense challenges. I now feel at peace with all that has happened.

During my pregnancy, I never lost sight of targets to aim for. I always had specific goals to work toward. These goals helped me survive the rough times. Going through this crisis helped me formulate further goals in subsequent years that related to my ultimate career in social work.

Pregnancy does not have to force you to drop out of school. Education was one of my priorities, and it was my self-determination that helped me find a way to complete my schooling. I completed the 10th grade at the group home with the help of individual tutors and classes in liaison with my school. I did not lose the school year and returned to school the following September. It was difficult facing people after being absent for some months. After completing high school, I went on to qualify for a social service certificate and then earned a bachelor's degree in social work. Later, I earned a master's degree in social work.

I am often asked if this crisis in my life led to my career in social work. This evidently was a major influence because it was only through this experience that I became aware of the social work profession. Until then, I had had no idea of the existence of social workers or of their roles. I had a positive relationship with my social worker. Perhaps this was somewhat related to the fact that I had already chosen to place my baby for adoption before I met her.

Other girls at the group home had negative experiences with social workers and felt pressured to relinquish their babies for adoption. I was able to see social workers at both ends of the spectrum. Some were sensitive to the girls' needs, and others were not there as supports for the girls. It was this lack of sensitivity in some of the social workers that initially motivated me to look into social work as a career. I can only hope that this thought always remains close at hand so that my sensitivity and genuineness as a social worker do not diminish as the years go by.

Many individuals enter helping professions after experiencing a personal crisis of some nature. It is important to work through this crisis and understand it in relation to why you desire to be in a helping role. If you have not dealt with the crisis in your life, you may carry issues around with you that will affect how you react to individuals you are working with. If you are overly sensitive about an issue, it may influence you to react in a way that may not be helpful to another person. You may react strongly to clients because of your own unresolved feelings. Your issues may not be their issues at all. This is just a word of caution: Work through your own issues if you are considering a career in a helping role in the future, or you may not be as helpful to your clients as you might think.

Closing Thoughts

This book has been prepared to help you during a difficult time in your life. Yet at the same time, it could be invaluable for those around you to read. Those people who care about you might develop a keener awareness of and sensitivity to your needs. Other teenagers who have never been pregnant may find this information useful in preventing pregnancy. You may have friends who are adopted teenagers and are struggling with questions about their birthparents. Through reading this book, they may develop an understanding about the pregnant teenager, which might assist them in resolving their concerns about their own birthparents.

By now you will realize that you are not alone. Some problems are common to all pregnant teenagers. Along the way, I have shared my personal thoughts and experiences with you so that you might find my comments hold some meaning for you. Others have generously shared their experiences to offer various perspectives and alternatives. Those who related their decisions and how they coped did it in the hope that it might assist you in understanding your options more fully so you can arrive at your own decision. These experiences of others and my experience were not intended to create any bias toward a particular option. None of the choices are easy, just different.

Now it is up to you to take control of your life and the decision you make. It is time for you to harness your own strength and determination and gather your supports to make the best of this dilemma in your life. The decisions that you make now will affect many areas of your life today and in the future. Whatever decision you make, you should realize the importance of thinking it through so that you are as sure as you can be that this is the right decision for you at this time. Above all, remember that you are a worthwhile person and have the ability to gain something positive from this crisis.

My hope is that as you have read this book you have done some self-exploration and discovered something new or reframed some existing ideas. The process I had to go through to enable me to write this book led me to further self-discovery, which is all part of working through the unfinished business of my own teenage pregnancy. You may retain various feelings about this event in your life for a long time to come. Your feelings about your pregnancy will not disappear overnight, and the experience may always remain a sensitive subject for you.

As I am a social worker, it is easy for me to feel that I should have all the answers for myself and should have all these issues dealt with and put aside on a neat shelf somewhere by now. This is not reality—social workers and other professionals are subject to the same feelings that other human beings have.

I hope that you found the message that social workers and other professionals are people underneath their professional exterior and they can be sensitive to your needs. The negative stereotype of the social worker, especially in the child welfare field, is well known. But there are capable and incapable people in all lines of work, so don't give up if you have a negative experience with one worker.

Writing this book has been an intense and emotional experience for me. I have learned and discovered as I have written, and the process has helped me put my mind at rest in many areas and has left me with a sense of peace.

To put my thoughts down on paper, I have had to rethink and relive the past. Some of the ideas that I have set down here I have not thought about in a very long time, but my energy has been channeled into a product that may be of use to other teenage girls faced with the problems I faced years ago.

Appendix A

Experiences of Others

The experiences of Debbie, Jon, and Lori are told in their own words. As youth, they experienced pregnancy or fatherhood and made different decisions. They describe what they faced and how they coped. Their stories are not intended to promote one decision over another but just to show the diversity in people's experiences.

Debbie

Debbie is 22 years old and is a single parent. She works for a Neighborhood House in British Columbia. She is a First Nation's outreach worker who works with families. The following is Debbie's story about her experience of teenage pregnancy and abortion.

When I was 15 years of age, I lived on my own in a rooming house. I had a kitchen and a bedroom on the second floor. I had been living on my own from the time I was 12 years of age. I was kicked out of my parents' home and never returned. I saw my parents once in a while. I lived on the street for a long time. I lived in party houses, on floors, in cars, on boats—wherever I could find a place to sleep. I didn't have very much. I think I owned a couple pairs of jeans, a few blouses, and a jacket.

From the age of 13, I was trying to become pregnant. I wanted someone I could love and someone who would love me back. This thought was always there either consciously or subconsciously. I became pregnant at 15.

I went to a health clinic to see if I was pregnant and to find out how far along I was. I was two months pregnant. The doctor assumed that I wanted an abortion, and this scared me. I didn't want an abortion. I wanted to keep my child. Social workers, my parents, and other people kept telling me that I shouldn't keep my baby. People threatened to take my baby away from me because I was so young. One night when I was coming home on the bus, I noticed a poster from an agency. I phoned this lady, and she said that no one could make me give up my child for adoption.

When I was first pregnant, I lived in a two-room basement suite. I was paying more than half my welfare in rent. Just before I had the baby, I moved to another two-room suite, and the rent was even more. This left me with very little to live on and to provide nutrition for the baby and myself. So I was put on a program called Healthiest Babies Possible. A lady phoned me, and she took me shopping. We bought cheese, lots of pork and beans, and lots of oranges. I lived off that for a long time.

When I was about six months pregnant, I finally went to the doctor because I didn't know what was going to happen. I had no idea about childbirth. I didn't go to prenatal classes because I assumed they would take my baby. I didn't seek help from anyone because of this fear.

When I was eight months and a week pregnant, my water broke while I was having a water fight with my neighbor. I couldn't understand why I was getting wet. I had no idea. I kept changing clothes until I had no clothes to change into. Then I phoned downstairs to a friend to ask if I could borrow some pants from her. She asked me why, and I told her that I kept getting wet. She said, "Oh no!" Then she explained that I was going to have my baby. I started crying because I didn't know what to expect. She told me that it was okay, and said that it was not as hard as everyone made it out to be. I resented her when I went into labor because it was hard, and it hurt. I couldn't understand why it was so painful.

In the hospital, they gave me some Demerol. I became so high that I didn't remember much of the childbirth. All I remember was telling the doctor off because I didn't like what he was doing. I didn't like him touching me. I was really naïve and nobody filled me in. I didn't talk to anyone because I thought everybody was out to take away my baby. Just from one social worker saying that my baby could be taken away from me, this built in a fear that I retained until my child was 4 or 5 years old. But it is a fear that I sometimes still have.

In the hospital, there was one nurse that I really liked and who really liked me. She was understanding, and she supported me through the time I was there. The other staff I found to be cold. They judged me from the time I was admitted. When I left the hospital, this nice nurse gave me some roses. This really made me feel good. She told me that she knew I could do it and that just gave me the little encouragement I needed.

After delivery, my baby had yellow jaundice and had to be placed in an incubator. The day I was to come home, staff told me that my baby couldn't come home for a few days. They didn't explain to me what jaundice was, and all I did was cry. I thought that my baby was going to die because I took some acid when I was first pregnant. I thought that I had caused her illness and feared that I could have killed my own child. I went through all these emotions, and I had nobody there to talk to or just to fill me in. Just before my baby was taken out of the incubator, her hair was standing up because of the heat and that made me laugh. I knew then that she was okay.

My baby was a big girl who weighed six pounds, nine ounces. I breastfed her and started her on soft food early to make sure she was healthy. During this time, the only support I had was from my sister, Roseanne. She was the only one who told me to keep my baby and who said that she would help me. She couldn't be there for me all the time because she lived in a logging camp. She only came into town every 6 or 12 months. I wrote to her, and that was one way for me to deal with things. She would write me back and would phone me if she thought it was important.

The baby's father never really spent time with me. He was an alcoholic and was always out drinking with his friends. He was 18 years old. Mentally he was 15, and I was 18. I grew up very quickly. I had no choice. He lived with me for a while, but he worked out of town. I hardly ever saw him. We would talk on the phone once in a while. I'd ask him how he was doing, and he'd say fine. He'd ask how the baby was and that was as far as it went. We were never really close. I used him to get pregnant and to have my child because that was what I wanted. I also used him to have a place to live, rather than sleeping outside.

My own determination helped me get through everything. I was going to prove to everybody that I could be the mother everyone thought I couldn't be. The more people pushed and said that I couldn't do it, the more I fought. People didn't believe that I could be a mother, and I showed them that I could cope with motherhood.

My only supports were my sister and the nurse in the hospital. But the nurse worked three shifts out of the five days of my hospitalization. I had a welfare worker, but I avoided her a lot. I was so afraid that the authorities were going to take my child away that I never let her know how I was really feeling. I appeared to be the good mother, and I was a good mother. But I was unable to share any difficulties I did have with her. I felt that she would assume that I would become an abusive mother. I was abused as a child and statistics show that people who have been abused as children abuse their children. I thought that she would want to remove my baby before any abuse could occur. I guess I must have had a lot of love to have been able to counteract the abuse cycle.

One of the messages I would pass on to pregnant teenagers is to find support. You need to make sure that you have people around you who understand what you are going through and can support you. I had no one to support me or to show me how to cope with my problems. So I ended up crying and feeling really depressed most of the time. It's not worth it. Just make sure that you have other resources to turn to.

Family members need to try to understand what their teenagers are going through. Regardless of what the girl's decision is, families need to be there for them. It is really important to teenagers to have love, respect, and understanding from their parents. If the parents can't understand their teenagers, the family should go for counseling. Pregnant teenagers are going to have a rough time ahead of them. To be told how dumb you are, how you shouldn't have done that, it's your own fault, or you made your bed, now lie in it, is not helpful. That kind of attitude just makes the teenagers resent their parents.

Often pregnant teenagers feel like giving their babies up for adoption and just killing themselves. I felt that way, and a lot of people I know and some of the people I work with feel that way. So parents should be there for their children.

I have known my youth worker since I was 12 years old. She was someone I could go to and yell at if I wanted to. She was great at times, but she didn't want me to have the child. She was one of the first people who told me to have an abortion. She said she would make arrangements to have my baby taken away from me. I would have preferred her to be understanding and tell me that it was my choice. I wish she'd said, "Here are the alternatives, and here is what you can do." I wish she'd filled me in on abortion, adoption, and childbirth. I wish social workers would take a similar role. Social workers should not play the heavies and indicate that they are the boss who says, "This is how it's done, and you've got to do it." I needed to know what my options were, because I didn't know. I think if I had known what was involved with each alternative, I might have changed my mind. If I had known what raising children would be like, then I think I would have changed my mind. With all the responsibility of having to do everything myself, it gets really rough.

When I had children, I stopped chumming around with my school friends. I had quit school, and I was returning to school when I became pregnant. I gave up on everything just to be the perfect mother and to be there for my child when she needed me. I ended up being all alone with no family, no friends, and no supports. I guess deep down I mistrusted my friends, too. I thought that maybe they would go to someone and say, "She's not doing a good job raising her children."

By the time I was 18 years old, I had a 2-year-old and a 1-year-old. I became pregnant again and decided that it would be too hard for me to raise three children. I knew I couldn't cope with another child so I decided to have an abortion.

This time it was different. My mother and father backed me up on this decision. They came over and helped me out a lot. They brought me to the hospital. After the abortion, my mother stayed overnight for two days to watch the children and helped with the housework so that I could get back on my feet. At that time, abortion was the best decision I could have made.

I went to see my doctor and went through the pregnancy test. He made all the arrangements. I went into the hospital in the morning and was out by three o'clock. Immediately afterward, I had an IUD inserted so that I could not get pregnant again.

I wasn't prepared for what was going to happen at the hospital. I didn't know anything about abortions. In the morning, they gave me a needle and made sure that I didn't eat or drink anything. I had general anesthesia. All I remember is the room spinning and someone saying count backwards from 10 while the IV was put in. I don't remember past the number nine.

When I awoke I felt disoriented. I'd forgotten where I was and what I was doing there. I felt tired and sick to my stomach. I felt sore, and my stomach felt knotted. Emotionally I felt really bad because I felt that I'd killed a baby. Later I thought about it and realized that it was the best decision for me, as I knew that I couldn't have coped with another child.

After the abortion, I had no one to share my thoughts with. Nobody talked about the abortion, but the thought stuck in my mind. My family helped with the practical side but not with the emotional side. Once in a while I still think about it, usually in September, as that was the month the baby would have been born.

I wish that I had been told about the abortion procedures beforehand, along with what I might expect to feel afterward. Then I would have looked for some support. I was not prepared for the afterthoughts, and it would have been easier if I'd been prepared. I thought it was simple and thought it would all be gone and would not bother me. But you find out differently after the abortion.

After the abortion I was very vulnerable. I had no friends, so I began drinking. Drinking was a way I could meet people and come out of my shell. I was unsure of myself and drinking gave me self-confidence. I enjoyed myself and had friends for the first time. I'd go out a couple of nights a week, and it got to the point where I couldn't stop after just a couple of drinks. One time I came home and my daughter thought that I was going to die because I was so sick. Then I knew that I had to stop drinking because I was hurting my children.

At that time I was living common law and our relationship was shaky. We had our differences, and we both drank. I went to Alcoholics Anonymous, and I learned how to cope with situations. It was a learning process for me. I made friends and opened up about some things that I was having a hard time dealing with.

Around this time I also joined an organization called Project Parent. This happened through a social worker from welfare who came over to my home and checked my children and my house. He checked my cupboard and fridge. He referred me to Project Parent and said I would meet other single mothers there. He thought this would be helpful for me, but I was really offended by this as it was three days before my welfare check was to be issued.

That was how I became involved in Project Parent. Actually I learned a lot there about children and the growing process and how to handle temper tantrums. It was a good support for me. I felt safe there and was able to open up in their groups. I allowed myself to cry in front of people for the first time.

Between Alcoholics Anonymous and Project Parent, I came a long way. I was 21 when I became pregnant with my son Nathan. I hadn't had a drink for one and one-half years and decided I was going to keep this baby. I had decided that if the fellow I was living with didn't like the idea, he could leave, as I was going to do it anyway. I'd been living with him for a year and a half. We had decided to go our own ways already, but we kept delaying the separation.

This pregnancy was easier. Having a man come to the hospital with me made me feel more self-assured. When I left the hospital this time, my common-law husband's mother looked after my two eldest children for a few hours while I got organized. My common-law spouse, Allen, was at home to greet me, and people came over to see the baby. It was as though everybody wanted to participate and wanted to cuddle the baby. That was so different from the time when I was alone after the first and second births. I could feel all the love, whereas the other times I didn't feel that. Even though my relationship with Allen wasn't the greatest, it was still better than being on my own.

Now I am a single parent with three children, and it is a great responsibility. I work, and my children attend a day care center. I have to do the housework, daily chores, and shopping, look after the children, and work. I have to survive on the amount of money I earn at work after paying all the bills. Often I'm just skimping along.

When the children are sleeping I find some time for myself, which is often about 10:30 at night. I usually go out on Thursday and Saturdays while my youngest son's father babysits. That's really nice for me and helps me to cope with things, as I don't have to worry about the children or babysitters.

My parents remain distant and do not babysit the children. That has not changed from the time I left home at 12. I'm very defensive with them. When I'm with them I have my guard up all the time because I don't know what they are going to say.

About a year ago, I returned to school. I took a course to be a family worker. On the weekends I did my homework or investigated resources in the community to see what services they provided. I graduated as an "A" student, and that was the first time for me. It felt really good. I was amazed that I could actually do something like that. It helped build my strength and my self-esteem.

Jon

Jon is 35 years old. He works as an auto body repairman. When he was a teenager, his girlfriend, Mary, became pregnant. Jon and Mary chose to marry as a way to deal with the pregnancy. Like Debbie, Mary also experienced abortion, which she had after having two children. Jon reflects on this experience and shares it with us here.

When I was 18 years old and my girlfriend, Mary, was 15 years old, I found out that she was pregnant. Our final decision was to get married rather than give the baby up for adoption or have an abortion. It was a difficult decision to make, but there was pressure from everyone to get married. At that time a marriage was considered the most socially acceptable alternative. My eldest sister kept saying, "Get married, get married." My parents felt we should get married. My girlfriend was leaning toward marriage. I kept changing my mind right up until the last minute. Once we married I decided to try to make the best of our situation.

We married when Mary was four or five months pregnant. She gave birth to a baby girl, and we named her Pam. I felt that we had made the right decision in keeping the baby. I don't regret the decision, because I now have a lovely daughter.

When I think back I realize that I never really understood, or even had the capacity to understand, what marriage really entailed. It was a bigger decision that I had thought at the time. Sometimes I feel that Mary should have had an abortion. But then I realize that I would not have my daughter Pam, whom I care for so much.

But I was not ready for marriage. It was really rough after we were married. Beforehand we had had support, but afterward we were totally on our own. Mary had support from the people at the group home where she had lived. Her parents had split up and were later divorced. The social workers were good supports to us prior to our marriage. They told us that if marriage was the decision we were going to make then that was great as far as they were concerned. Unfortunately, they did not continue that support after we were married.

Mary's uncle helped us out. The bit of support we had came from the older people and not from people our own age. We couldn't seem to relate to anyone our own age any more, so we had to associate with older people. Mary seemed to handle this better than I did. All our friends were still in school. I lost all my friends, and Mary lost a lot of her friends for the next three to four years.

The first couple of years were really tough for both of us. We went through a lot of changes. I didn't have the chance to do the things the other teenagers did. I stopped maturing. I couldn't grow up the way I feel I should have. I had to become an instant adult.

We lived in my parents' basement suite for a year and a half. We had a difficult time coping with life, but this living arrangement helped us initially. If we hadn't lived there, we wouldn't have been able to survive.

I didn't even know what sort of job to look for. I had to quit school in the middle of the 11th grade to take a job as an apprentice boatbuilder. It was not the job I wanted, but it was work. The trade was better than nothing, as I hadn't finished high school.

Once I was working, I could no longer hang around with the other teenagers. It was as if I didn't fit in with this crowd anymore. Yet I didn't seem to fit in with the fellows at work either, as they were in their mid-20s, 30s, and older. This made for a lonely existence, and I ended up drinking in order to be socially accepted by the older guys. Alcohol helped me to overcome my feelings of insecurity and made me feel more mature. I could be accepted as one of the boys when I drank with them. Sadly though, it only added further problems in my life, as I became an alcoholic.

Three years later we had another child named Sean. Mary was 18 years old then. Shortly after Sean's birth, Mary became pregnant again. This time we decided on abortion because we already had two children and could not support a third. We were still too young. My wife was not even 19 years old and already had two children.

The abortion was so easy. Mary just went into the hospital one day and then she was home. But the idea bothers me when I look at pictures of my two children and think that there might have been another child. There is not much I can do about it now, so I've had to let go of these thoughts. Today my thinking is different. I now believe that we shouldn't have decided on abortion, but I can't condemn myself because at the time it was the best decision we could have made.

I spent many years searching for a satisfying job. I completed the boat-building apprenticeship. I worked at different jobs, including assistant manager of an IGA store, sales, union president of a local, and operator of a cabaret. I completed another apprenticeship in carpentry. By the age of 29, I'd completed a third apprenticeship as an auto body repairman. I never knew where "Jon" belonged. I was always searching for something outside of myself. Today I am satisfied with myself and now feel that I can go after whatever I want in life. I have more self-confidence. I've always been a striver, and I haven't given up yet.

But it took me a long time to get to this point. It makes me realize my immaturity at the time of our marriage. When I look at my 16-year-old daughter, it is hard for me to believe that Mary and I were married at her age. I keep thinking that we must have been older, but we weren't.

It seems as though we made such a wrong decision. At the ages of 18 and 15, our marriage didn't have a chance of lasting.

But our marriage did last for eight years. Many of my friends were married in their teenage years. They are all divorced now. I'm not implying that this happens to everyone who marries young, but I think that if you get married just because of pregnancy it is totally the wrong reason. You are still too young to really understand the full implications of marriage and sharing a life together intimately.

Intimacy demands being able to let each other be yourself. I was not able to be myself in the marriage. Whatever Mary wanted I would do because I didn't know any other way. I think that a number of people are like that when they are that age. We didn't know what we wanted or needed in our relationship.

Today Mary and I are divorced. She is remarried, and her life is going along fairly well. I just pray that it will continue that way. Today Mary and I can be friends. I've learned to realize that I do love her. I have no bad feelings and no animosity toward her. She is a lovely women and a good mother. My two children—Sean age 13 and Pam age 16—live with her.

I now have a daughter who is growing up. I just hope that she never has to go through a similar experience. It gets difficult now that I'm thinking through everything again as I watch my daughter become a teenager. I don't know how I would handle it if she came walking through the door and said that she was pregnant. What would I suggest to her?

When I was going through the experience, I didn't have anyone to share it with. I would hope that if teenagers do decide to marry that they keep seeking help after their marriage.

I don't regret what happened. It was a good learning experience in spite of everything. During the process I became a member of Alcoholics Anonymous. This organization helped me turn a lot of my mind around. I also became a Christian, which provided me with guidance and support. This firm belief system gave me a better understanding of what life is all about. I don't feel alone now. Religion may not be right for everyone, but it was very helpful to me.

I also completed a Christian counseling course, which added to my level of awareness. I hope that someday I might be able to help others who have had problems similar to those I've encountered. I hope that by sharing my experiences here others might not have to go through the difficulties that Mary and I went through.

Lori

Lori had an abortion at three and a half months into her pregnancy. Now she is 19 years old and is seven and a half months pregnant. This time she plans to keep her baby and take on the role of a single parent. Lori shares both of her experiences with us.

When I was 17 years old, I suddenly found myself pregnant. At that time I was working as a counter girl in a restaurant, I had left school in the 10th grade and had been out of school and living away from home for about a year. I shared a house with my boyfriend and two other friends. We were having a good time.

I discovered my pregnancy in early January and confronted my boyfriend with it. We discussed it and then told our parents. Then there was a big controversy. Everyone asked me what I wanted to do. But when I said that I wanted to keep the baby, everybody said, "No. That's not what you want to do because it's going to ruin your life and everybody's life." My boyfriend decided that I should have an abortion, but that was not what I wanted. That was what he wanted and what everybody else wanted. Nobody really took my feelings into consideration. That bothered me because it was happening to me and not to my boyfriend, not to his parents, and not my mom. I was given an ultimatum that I had to either do it their way or else leave. Both families said that they would have nothing to do with me unless I had an abortion. I figured that I should do as they wished and have the abortion.

I had to go through the whole ordeal of telling my employer and my friends that I was pregnant. I had to leave work to have the abortion because my boss wouldn't give me time off. He let me know that abortion was against his morals. He was a good Catholic with five children. That didn't seem fair to me. I felt that he was discriminating against me, so I decided that leaving work was the best thing to do.

It wasn't too hard telling my friends because everybody knew that I had been living with my boyfriend for six months. Everybody knew who he was, and they figured that he was a nice guy. My friends assumed that I was going to keep the baby. They said that they would do all sorts of things to help. A lot of my friends turned their backs on me when I told them that I was going to have an abortion. My friends had urged me to keep the baby.

Two of my girlfriends were truly good. They listened to my point of view. They said that they would stick by me whatever my decision was. I respected that. They didn't say, "This is what we want you to do," or "Do it our way or we won't be your friends." Their friendship wasn't conditional. I needed that kind of support. But later when I needed support after the abortion, they weren't there. Some of my friends didn't want to talk to me because they were angry with me for having an abortion. It took them about six months to realize that an abortion had been best for me at that time.

When I went into the hospital to have the abortion, I was three and one-half months pregnant. There was the pressure of time. I was told that I would have to have it then or never. I knew that if I waited any longer I would have to have an abortion by induced labor. My cousin had had a late abortion and she didn't recommend it. I knew that if I were going to have an abortion, I would have to have it immediately. We had already spent a lot of time discussing the decision back and forth. The time went by quickly.

I might have decided myself to have an abortion if I had had the time to think about it instead of having had everybody decide for me. I felt trapped. First of all, I cancelled the abortion three days before I was supposed to go into the hospital and refused to see the doctor. I thought I would do it my way. It was then that I was given the ultimatum. I had to do it their way or get out of their lives. I was living with my boyfriend. He literally told me that if I were going to have the baby, I would have to pack my bags and leave. His parents said that they would have nothing to do with the baby and me. They said, "Don't come looking for us six months down the line asking for support, because we are not going to give it to you."

I eventually did have the abortion. The day before the abortion I went in to see my doctor to have laminaria tents inserted. I didn't know what this was, and I really didn't care. They told me that the laminaria tents would absorb the mucus from my uterus and cause my cervix to expand. The doctor left me sitting in the examining room for 40 minutes. I didn't even want to be there in the first place, so they were lucky that I didn't leave. But I knew that if I didn't do it everybody else's way, I'd be stuck. So I did what I had to do.

At first there was no discomfort from the laminaria tents. By the time I got home I felt menstrual-like cramps. I had a hot shower to alleviate the pain. I used hot water bottles and pain killers and had a restless sleep. I had to get up at 6:30 A.M. to get ready to go to the hospital. I had been advised to wear something loose in order to be comfortable afterward.

After they admitted me to day surgery, my boyfriend was asked to leave. I said that I should like to have him sit with me for a while, but they said no. It would have made me feel better to have had him keep me company for the two hours that I had to wait. They escorted me down the corridor to a locker room where they told me to take off my clothes and put on a surgical gown and stockings. They took a blood sample. A nurse weighed me. At 9:00 A.M., they gave me an IV. I was taken to a room with four other girls who were there for abortions. I was the last one to go into the operating room. It was like an assembly line. But I was a person, not an object.

Nobody took the time to explain what was about to happen. I didn't see the doctor until 11:30 A.M. I found the nurses very cold. They paid no attention to my feelings or to the feelings of the other girls in the room.

It was 11:20 when I was wheeled into the OR [operating room]. There was a nurse, an anesthetist, a doctor, and an intern. They slid me off the stretcher and onto a metal table. I was told to close my eyes and was given a needle. The doctor came in and said, "I'm hungry. I want to go to lunch after this." I said, "You're not going anywhere. I'm here for one reason, so get it done with. I'm hungry too!" They didn't let me eat for 24 hours before surgery.

I was given a second needle, and the next thing I remember was waking up in the recovery area and looking at the clock. It was 12:50. A few minutes later I was up and walking around. Everyone else who had gone into surgery before me was still in bed. I wanted to get in and out of there as quickly as possible.

I remember one girl sitting there and being so proud of herself for having had the abortion. She had a 6-month-old baby at home and had become pregnant again accidentally. She didn't want the second child and babbled on about how much better she felt now, after the abortion. I thought that she must have been crazy because I felt as though I had lost something when I left the hospital.

I sat there until 1:30 P.M., when my boyfriend came to get me.

When I got home, I was so glad it was over. Physically I felt terrible. I felt like all my energy had been drained. I was hungry. I didn't really want to do anything but eat and sleep. I felt like a hangover. About midnight, the cramps became painful. I woke up to find myself alone. My boyfriend had told me that he would stay with me for the duration of that day, but he had figured that once midnight rolled around he could take off. I woke up in a frenzy. I was afraid that I was going to bleed to death. I didn't understand what was happening.

We had moved into the apartment block only two weeks before, and I didn't know anyone. I felt lost, confused, and hurt. I started crying and phoning people. Nobody appreciated it when I phoned late at night looking for my boyfriend. I left a message with a friend to tell him that I had gone home to my mom's house. I got dressed and was planning to take the bus. It was 2:00 A.M. and raining. I could hardly walk. I stood at the bus stop, and then my boyfriend drove up and took me home. I only wanted to be somewhere with other people.

In the beginning, everybody had told me that I might stay with them after the abortion. When I woke up with nobody there, I was scared. When I needed them, they weren't there. It took me a long time to regain my trust in my family and friends. I needed emotional support and without it I felt lost. I did a lot of thinking during that period of time about who my real friends were. I had a lot of doors slammed in my face. I had to cope with things on my own. Even my boyfriend didn't seem to understand what I was feeling.

Until recently I didn't realize what my boyfriend was feeling either. He felt like he wasn't the center of attention. Everything was happening to me. He felt that I was ignoring him. He didn't realize the changes that I was going through. We neglected each other's feelings, and this led to a break-up in our relationship six weeks later. I hadn't look deeply enough into how others around me were feeling and reacting. I hadn't realized that my boyfriend had had feelings too, and that he had felt hurt.

Now I am 19 years old, and I am seven and one-half months pregnant. The same fellow is the father of this baby. We still see each other on and off, but have not lived together since the separation following the abortion. This time I plan to keep the baby.

I plan to go back to school in the fall and complete the 12th grade. Tupper High School has a special program for teenage mothers, and they offer day care at the school. My baby will be 5 months old by then.

Until last month I lived with my mom in her house. Then I moved into the suite on the ground level of the same house. One of my girl-friends will soon be moving in with me. I have decided that I need my own space because I like to have my friends over, and it's awkward with my mom around. I had been used to living on my own for two years and all of a sudden I felt confined. My mom doesn't bug me, and I don't bug her. When there's a problem, my mom is close by upstairs. That will be handy when I go into labor. I won't have to go looking for somebody. I won't have to worry about being alone. I also have a roommate. I need that security.

My mom's initial reaction to this second pregnancy was that she didn't want me being pregnant in her house, bearing an illegitimate child. She didn't want my little brother subjected to this. She didn't want her friends to know. In the beginning she didn't even think about me. She thought about how everybody else was going to react. She had the same initial reaction this time that she had had with my first pregnancy. She did not think about how I was going to cope with my pregnancy. It is not my mom who is pregnant and has to face her friends, it's me. The funny thing is that now the whole family has accepted my pregnancy. Nobody has turned their backs on me. Even my grandmother thinks it's great.

I have a 13-year-old brother who lives with my mom and a half-brother and half-sister who live with my dad. My mom told me that my younger brother ran around the school saying, "I'm going to be an uncle." He finds it hard to deal with the fact that I'm going to be a mother because he and I used to play around a lot before I was pregnant. He is himself a teenager, and he is going through a lot of changes too. So we are both changing.

This time I have all kinds of emotional support. I have my family, social workers, and doctors. I have people I can trust and that is a great help. A year ago I asked what others wanted me to do. I took their advice and now regret it. I've done a lot of growing up during this last year.

When I was four months pregnant, I ended up in the hospital for five days. This was scary because I wasn't sure what was happening. I had been visiting my boyfriend, and on my way home I started bleeding. I went to my doctor, but he wasn't in. Eventually I was admitted into the hospital. I bled for a day and a half and was confined to bedrest for 36 hours. They placed me in a gynecology ward. I felt out of place as other women were there to have abortions, among other reasons. This hospital didn't have an obstetrics ward.

The rest of my pregnancy went well with the exception of poor weight gain. I had two ultrasounds. Before having an ultrasound, I was asked to drink a lot of liquid and was not to go to the washroom for two hours. This is pretty hard to do even when you're not pregnant. They took a machine with a microphone and ran it up and down my stomach. It is computerized and sound waves determine the size and location of the fetus. When I saw the fetus on the screen, it just looked like a shape.

During my pregnancy, a health nurse and nutritionist visited me every two weeks at home under a program called Healthiest Babies Possible. They checked my weight gain and calorie intake. They provide food vouchers for people on a low income. Basically they provided support.

I also attend a program for single pregnant teenagers right now called REACH. The youngest girl I met there had a baby at 13. I thought, "How can a child raise a child?" I know I'm young, and I'll find it difficult at 19. Part of me feels that if you are old enough to get pregnant then you are old enough to look after the baby. But this girl wasn't any older than my little brother, and it really made me think. It's scary now for me to think of having a baby around all the time, but I know that I can handle it. By going to places like REACH, I saw girls who think of babies as dolls. One girl said, "If my baby is fat and bald I'm not going to keep it." These programs for teenagers are trying to help girls realize that babies are real, and the workers give you a lot of support.

I am going to begin prenatal classes at the health unit six weeks before my baby is due. They will teach me breathing exercises and discuss labor and delivery. It is only nine weeks before my baby is due, but

I find it hard to think that far ahead. I can deal with things more easily if I think about them in small segments and take time to think everything through.

At present I'm collecting unemployment insurance benefits. These benefits will last until the end of March. Then I will be eligible for public assistance. Once my roommate moves in, this will help with expenses. I spoke to my social worker, and she said that once I am collecting income assistance, I will be able to get financial aid to help me buy some of the items I'll need for the baby, such as a crib.

If I could pass on something from my own experience to other pregnant teenagers, it would be to tell them that they should be sure that the decision they make is their own. It is their pregnancy and no one else's. They should take their own feelings into consideration, think through their own decision, and consider how their decision will affect them later on. There are many variables that will change over time. I've had to accept that what has happened to me has happened. It is in the past, so I can't change that fact now.

Appendix B

Suggestions

For Family

As parents of a pregnant teenager, your attitudes and reactions are immensely important. Your initial shock and disbelief may be equal to your daughter's. Your feelings will be transmitted to your daughter in one way or another. Even if you do not tell her directly and even if you try to disguise your reactions, she will know you well enough to ascertain your real feelings. How you respond to her condition will affect how she adjusts to her pregnancy. She will reflect your own adjustment to it. Your support may be just what she needs to help her through this experience.

It probably took all of your daughter's courage to tell you about her predicament in the first place. She may have feared your reaction and feared hurting you. She may have feared that you would disown her.

During this crisis, your daughter will be learning the skills of coping with problems. If she can learn to cope with her pregnancy, she will be able to use these skills to cope with other difficulties she will face in the future.

You may, as a parent, find yourself in a dilemma. You may realize that your child is now faced with an adult world and with adult decisions before she has herself grown up. You will want the easiest course for her, and you may want to make her decisions for her. She may even want you to decide for her because she may be confused. But your daughter must make her decision on her own because she will have to live with it for the rest of her life.

You can help your daughter by discussing all of the choices she has and by trying to keep an open mind. She may choose the course that you would not choose. If she makes her decision to please you rather than for her own benefit, she may later regret it and blame you for your influence.

Your reaction to her and to her problem may run the gamut from rejection to overprotection. Your disapproval might have a lasting impression on your relationship with your daughter in the years to come. The most helpful approach you can take is just to stand by your daughter, because she needs you now more than ever. Envision yourself in her place and think about how you might feel and react. Your relationship with your daughter during this crisis will be determined in part by the relationship that existed prior to her pregnancy.

Whether she decides to marry or live with a partner, to place the child for adoption, to become a single parent, or to terminate the pregnancy, she will still need your support. You will need to be there to comfort her without judging her and to assist her with practical and emotional matters. You can help to rebuild her self-confidence by letting her know that she is still the same girl whom you have always been proud of. You can reassure her that your love does not diminish when she finds herself in difficulty.

She may fluctuate between needing a shoulder to cry on and asserting herself as an adult. She may be irritable and moody, or she may withdraw. For no apparent reason she may lash out in anger at those who are conveniently close at hand. Try not to take her anger personally because she may feel angry at the world.

Her pregnancy is not an isolated event. It will affect all of your family. Pretending that it does not exist will not make it go away. If your daughter decided to place her baby for adoption, you may wonder about the baby and may speculate what it would have been like if the baby had remained part of your family. You also will experience loss and grief.

You may even have the desire to raise this child yourself because your daughter still seems like a child to you. This grandchild may be very important to you, but if you get this urge, you should think it through carefully and talk it over thoroughly with your daughter. Think about whose needs you are attempting to meet. Are they your daughter's needs, the baby's needs, or your own needs? Grandparents who secretly raise the child of a daughter as if it were their own may add to family conflict and role confusion. If it is done openly, there is the best opportunity for success.

You may have strong negative feelings toward your daughter's boyfriend. Blaming him is not helpful to her. Conception requires two people. Angry feelings toward him may drive a wedge between your daughter and yourself. If you put pressure on her not to see her boyfriend, you may force her to choose between him and you. What if she chooses him? She may need you and her boyfriend for support. Your attempt to pressure her will only create a barrier between you. If she has to sneak behind your back to see him she cannot be honest with you. Her boyfriend may already feel responsible and blame himself. He may want to help to the extent that he can. If you force an end to the relationship, you may be denying your daughter a source of support. You must leave it up to her to decide whether she wants to continue to see her boyfriend.

Keep in mind that your dreams for your daughter need not be shattered. It will be difficult for your daughter no matter what decision she makes, but with your help she can make the best decision. You can help your daughter find out information about all the options. You can accompany her to agencies to talk with professionals if she wants this type of support. You can offer to go with her at the time of delivery or termination. Hugs, acceptance, and love do help.

For Boyfriends

Teenage love is a special relationship between two young people. You may have deep regard for your girlfriend, or your relationship may have been over before she discovered that she is pregnant. Regardless of the status of your relationship, you are the father of the child she is carrying, and she may well need your help now.

You may be emotionally closer to her than any other person is. You may be the first person she confides in about her pregnancy, or you may find out through someone else. It could be comforting to her to have you stand beside her and be there when she reaches out to you for a hug or a hand to hold. On the other hand, she may not want your support at all, and you may have to respect her wishes.

She may be confused about how she feels about you. Some days she may pull you close to her; other days she may push you away. She may not be sure what she wants right now. She may ask you to accompany her to the hospital or to the clinic.

Because of the effect upon you, you may have strong feelings about her decision. You will need to be fundamentally open and honest with her, and you should discuss the choices open to her. If you push her in one direction, it may well result in her pulling in the opposite direction. If she feels pressured by you to make a particular decision, she may later regret it and blame you. If she makes the decision that she believes will please you, she will be making it for the wrong reasons. Try to imagine yourself in her place and understand how you might feel if you were a girl with her problems. Try to understand her reasoning, her thoughts, and her feelings.

Her pregnancy is certain to affect your life in some way. The crisis may bring too much stress into your relationship for it to endure, and you may have to deal with ending the relationship. Or you may have had only a casual relationship and be angry at finding yourself caught up in a predicament. You may feel responsible for your girlfriend's predicament, and you may blame yourself. You may feel terrified of becoming a father at such a young age. You may feel pressured to marry her or live with her to "make it right." Whatever your condition, you may also have strong emotions. Your girlfriend may be too much in need of help herself at this time to listen to or help you with your needs. You may need to confide in someone to get it off your chest. Perhaps you have a best friend, a brother, or a sister. You may benefit from talking with your girlfriend's social worker or someone at a youth agency.

Your family will also be affected, as this is a potential grandchild to them. Do not underestimate the effect this will have on them, and remember to lean on them for support too.

For Friends

During teenage years, friends are of the utmost importance, and peer influence is stronger than at any other time in your life. If your friend becomes pregnant, she will need to be reassured that she has loyal friends. She will fear being an outcast. You can demonstrate to her that her friends will not judge her and will stick by her. You can act as her sounding board. Your reactions will have a tremendous effect on how she feels about herself and the decisions she makes.

Try not to give her advice. She could be getting advice from everyone. She may be feeling pushed and pulled by the attitudes of her parents, boyfriend, and social worker. It is important for you to remain impartial. Just a sensitive, nonjudgmental approach can be a great help because no one has a good answer for her now. She must make the ultimate decision about what is best for her. You can help her find out about all of her choices, and you can support her in whatever decision she makes. You may believe that she is making the wrong decision because it is not what you would do, but what is best for you is not necessarily best for her.

Try to avoid getting too emotionally entangled in your friend's problems. You must be objective if you want to help. If you get upset, it will only heighten her turmoil. She may then hesitate to confide in you for fear of upsetting you more. One good friend can be the most reliable support to a pregnant teenager. Your friend will need your help not only during her pregnancy, but afterward, when she is reestablishing her social life. Just accept her and stay friends with her throughout this time.

For Professionals

If you are a helping professional, sooner or later you will come into contact with a pregnant teenager. Facing you may be a frightened young lady suddenly confronting the need to make adult decisions of a highly emotional nature. She may feel ashamed, ambivalent, lonely, confused, frightened, and angry. She may appear flippant about her pregnancy and act as if she doesn't care, or she may take it very seriously. She may be acting out her angry feelings of "why me?" and may yell and scream at you. She may withdraw and not want to talk to anyone. Regardless of her outward behavior, remember that chances are, inside she is frightened. Even though resources are available to her, she must be willing to accept help from them. This places an increased burden on you to encourage her to use those resources.

She may fear you because you represent authority. She may fear that you have the power to take her baby away from her or that you will pressure her into doing something that she does not want to do. It is important that you make your role clear to her, because she may see all professionals as cast in the same mold. She may not know where to begin or even what questions to ask. You may have to take some risks and gently endeavor to find out what she might be going through and what she needs to know. She will need an unbiased explanation of options open to her.

You will need to let her know that you are not there to tell her what to do but to help her explore all the options open to her. Regardless of what you perceive to be her best interest, you can help her best by assisting her in arriving at her own decision. She must live with the decision, not you. You may find your position difficult because you have to consider the needs of the teenager as well as the needs of the unborn child. You may have a strong opinion as to what her decision should be, but pressure and threats will only serve to push her into a corner and away from you. She will be forced to retaliate, assert her independence, and try to prove that she is right. You will become locked into a power struggle with her and no one will win. You will lose her trust. She will no longer confide in you, even if she really needs your help. If she does give in to your point of view and decides under pressure, she will have the consequences of her decision to deal with later on. She may have guilt feelings and an emotional block.

Try to remember your own teenage years and realize how unequipped you would have been to deal with a crisis such as this. How would you have wanted those around you to react? Sensitivity, warmth, and genuineness are the key elements in your approach to her. If you are nonjudgmental, you will help her to preserve her self-worth. Remember the burdens of adolescence that she will be struggling with. This experience will only heighten her ambivalence about autonomy, dependence, independence, and sexuality. Part of her will want to remain a child who wants to be taken care of, whereas part of her will want to be a woman who asserts her independence. This struggle to develop her own identity may make it hard for her to ask for help.

You can play an important role during her pregnancy and afterward by helping her reflect on her experience and extract what she has learned. Although she may feel her world is falling apart right now, she will grow from this pain, and you can help her see the positive elements.

Maintaining your contact with her after her pregnancy is crucial, as this is often a time when everyone feels the crisis is past and pulls out their support. If she chooses to keep her baby, she will have increased responsibility and ongoing stress. She may need help in locating resources such as parent support groups, financial aid, or day care. If she has an abortion or places her baby for adoption, she will experience a loss and a natural grief reaction. In adoption, the process does not end for the birthparent when the adoption papers are signed. Sometimes this marks the beginning of another crisis as birthparents deal with the loss or try to bury their grief. She may need you most after her pregnancy when she is rethinking her decision and trying to integrate the experience into her present life.

You may need to offer counseling to the baby's father. He is often the forgotten link, although he may be equally troubled and confused. The pregnancy will have had an effect on his life and his family's life too. He may require assistance in preparing himself for a new role and increased responsibility.

The girl's family may need help in adjusting to her pregnancy. Their lives will also be affected by it. If you can find ways to support the family, your help will benefit the pregnant girl, because the family will then be able to become more sensitive to her needs and provide optimal support.

For Hospital Staff

A pregnant teenager who comes to the hospital, whether for an abortion or for delivery, is bound to be frightened and may be all alone. She will need as much sensitivity and kindness from the staff as possible. She will probably fear being judged by staff members. The manner in which you care for this patient will have a great effect on her. Teenagers seem to pick up instantly the attitudes and value judgments of those around them.

Teenagers often evoke strong negative feelings in adults. They may remind you of struggles you had as a teenager. Many staff members do not enjoy working with adolescents and perceive it as a struggle rather than as a challenge. If you find yourself being judgmental toward a pregnant teenager, use this as an indicator that your approach will not be helpful to this girl. Recognize which patients you work best with and ask to be reassigned to care for another patient.

The teenager deserves the respect given to all patients and will only be hurt by a punitive attitude. She probably judges herself more harshly than anyone else could. Remember that this girl is facing a difficult situation and has no easy answers. She feels vulnerable in the hospital and often reacts just as the child who needs comfort would react.

The adolescent is in transition between the child and the adult world and lacks the skills of the adult to deal with complex systems such as hospitals. She may never have been in the hospital before. She will be unsure about what will happen there and may feel too ashamed or afraid to ask. You should assume that she knows nothing and begin your explanations on that premise. This does not imply that you should talk down to the adolescent, however, as respect is a vital element in dealing with teenagers.

You should try to be sensitive to the girl's needs when you decide which room she is to occupy on your ward. If she is having an abortion or placing her child for adoption, you would be thoughtless to put her in a room with other mothers who are caring for their babies.

The teenager tends to delay telling anyone about her pregnancy. Time goes by, and when she decides to have an abortion, her pregnancy may be advanced. She may require a late abortion. This is bound to be a difficult experience for her, and she will need sensitive nursing staff who do not have strong prejudices against abortion. Younger teenagers are more likely to have late abortions than are older girls. The emotional effect of an abortion in late pregnancy seems to be greater than it is in early pregnancy.

The teenager in the hospital should be encouraged to have someone with her whether she is admitted for an abortion or for delivery. She may not have thought of this beforehand. You might be of assistance if there is anyone she would want to call. If she has no supportive family or friends able to be with her, perhaps your hospital has volunteers who can be a support. No one needs to be alone.

If a teenager has preexisting emotional problems, this should be a signal to you that she may be at high risk for further problems after the abortion or delivery. Pregnancy will only serve to compound any existing psychosocial problems. You could be helpful by envisioning her in the context of her environment and identifying any psychosocial problems that she might desire assistance with. You might make a referral to the hospital social worker to assess whether she requires support during her hospitalization or on discharge.

For Group Home Staff

Group homes are useful resources for the pregnant teenager. Pregnant teenagers, however, may be reluctant to use these services if they are planning to keep their babies, and more girls are keeping their babies these days. Some group homes for pregnant teens have the reputation of trying to steamroll their residents toward placing their babies for adoption. Girls may fear this bias. Group homes for pregnant teens need to address the needs of teenagers who plan to be mothers. Group homes should be available as resources to teenagers who are pregnant, regardless of the outcome of their pregnancy. Teenage mothers can benefit from having a place to return to after the delivery where they can learn the necessary skills to care for their child and where they can receive the emotional support they need at this time.

Group home staff may think that their roles have ended once the girl goes into the hospital, but the girl may need ongoing support after hospitalization. The group home staff might either provide follow-up support for residents to stay on for a while until they resettle, or they might refer the girl to other community resources.

Group home staff should also be sensitive to the girl's needs while she is in the hospital. Visits from staff might be comforting. She may just need to know that someone cares. If the girl is alone, perhaps another resident from the home might accompany her to the hospital and stay with her. It is likely that she has developed a close friendship with another resident. This resident might perform a valuable service in preparing the other girls for their own hospitalization and delivery.

For Volunteers

If you are a volunteer who works with pregnant teenagers, you will need to be aware of your own values and attitudes. You must be comfortable with teenage pregnancy so that you may discuss it openly and honestly.

You must be careful not to influence the girl into doing what you think is right. She is the only person who can decide what is best for her, and she must live with her decision. You will need to be a good listener, just like a close friend. She may need to lean on someone. You may be able to get closer to her than a professional person would because she may fear the authority of child welfare agencies and transfer this fear to all professionals. You can assist her in reflecting on her dilemma and in investigating all of her options.

You must try to avoid becoming too deeply enmeshed in her problems. If you lose all of your objectivity, you will not be as helpful to her as you could be. She will need someone who doesn't fall apart or get upset when she tells her story. If she feels that she is burdening you with her problems, then she may stop confiding in you. As you are outside her family circle, you might be able to get her to talk to you about her pregnancy in a less emotional way than a family member would. She is not tied to you with the strings of emotion.

As a volunteer, you might become a constant person in her life. You would be able to remain by her side through the whole ordeal and be there afterward. You might be a key person to assist her in identifying her own needs, and then you might direct her to appropriate community resources.

For Adopted Teenagers

Although this book is directed to the pregnant teenager, if you are an adopted teenager, you may discover something about yourself as you read and think. You may be struggling with your sense of personal identity and sense of yourself as an autonomous individual during your teenage years. This self-exploration often evokes thoughts and questions about your birthparents.

If you happen to be a teenager who is adopted and pregnant, you may find your problems are compounded. If you have not had these thoughts about your birthparents before, pregnancy may well precipitate these questions. Not only will you have to face the decisions about your pregnancy, but you may be overly sensitive to the adoption and separation issues. You may still be dealing with your perception that your birthmother rejected you, while at the same time you may be considering the alternative of adoption. You may also have thoughts about this baby being the first blood relative in your life, and so your decision about the pregnancy may take on a special meaning.

As an adoptee, you will be trying to make sense of these two sets of parents in your background. On the one hand, you have a mom and a dad who have been parents to you as you have grown up. On the other hand, the reality is that there are two birthparents out there somewhere, including the mother who gave birth to you. It is a natural process to wonder about the unknown elements of your heredity and identity.

You may fear opening up these topics with your adoptive parents for fear of hurting them. Maybe neither you nor your parents will approach the subject for varying reasons. Each of you may wait for the other to take the initiative. This could be a loss for both of you. If you are able to talk about your adoption, it could prove to be a valuable experience and strengthen your adoptive family by getting rid of barriers and enriching your relationships.

Not all adoptees, however, have strong needs to talk about their adoption, just as not all adoptive parents can deal with their questions easily. Your parents have sensitive areas too. Questions about birthparents may touch on many areas that are difficult for your parents to discuss. They may generate feelings of inadequacy, if your adoptive parents were unable to bear children, or they may raise other concerns. Parents have different capacities as to what they can handle emotionally, and they may have had no preparation to know how to respond to your questions and needs.

If you were adopted, it is very likely that your birthmother was a pregnant teenager. I hope that you can gain an understanding of the pregnant teenager and the dilemma she is faced with. She has no easy answers, just as your birthmother had no easy solution to her problems. Think about how you might feel if you were pregnant right now. What decisions would you make and why? How would you feel? Would you be scared? Your birthmother tried to make the best of a very difficult situation. If you are able to imagine what it might have been like to be in her shoes, then you may be able to come to terms with some of your feelings and doubts about your own adoption.

Appendix C

The Adoption Triangle

doption is a lifelong relationship between the mother who relinquishes her child for adoption, the child, and the adopting parents. They form the adoption triangle. If you are considering placing your child for adoption, you will need to be aware that your feelings for your baby will not vanish magically once the adoption is complete. This is a misconception that many teenagers have been encouraged to believe. People may have told you that once the adoption is over, you will not think about it again. You may give up your rights in adoption, but you do not give up your feelings.

It would be highly unusual if you went through this experience and never thought about your child again. It is likely you will wonder if your child is okay. You may hope that your child will understand why you placed him or her for adoption, and you will hope that the child does not feel rejected. You will wonder what he or she looks like. You may wonder if your child thinks about you and what the adoptive parents have told him or her about you. Your child will always occupy a special place in your heart, and you will think of your child on his or her birthdays. Over time, as you grow into adulthood and have subsequent pregnancies, you will likely think even more about this first pregnancy and the child you relinquished.

Placing a baby for adoption is a loss that is not acknowledged by society. The grief process is usually private. Some people keep their grief buried rather than deal with the pain of the loss, but it does not go away on its own. Some birthmothers note that their interest in their child actually increases over time, even though the acute distress diminishes. Those who later experience adoption reunion can be flooded by many feelings of loss that were never dealt with at the time of the adoption.

Adoption is a serious decision. You will need to consider the long-term consequences. This may be the furthest thing from your mind right now, but you are bound to think about it later. You will need to prepare yourself for the aftermath of adoption and the effects it may have on you in the years to come.

Adoptions can be confidential, that is, closed, or can vary in the degree of openness. You can be given identifying information or even meet the adoptive parents. Regardless of whether you choose open or closed adoption, adoption records may be accessible to adult adoptees.

The need that some adoptees have to find out about their roots is especially important during adolescence when they are searching to find their own sense of personal identity. This compounds the struggles for identity that are common to all teenagers. Knowing our past provides us with the sense of ourselves that we have today. Some adoptees have little curiosity about their birthparents. Some desire further information about them and about the circumstances of their adoption. Others are driven to search for those parents. Those who decide to search for their birthparents have a long, intense struggle ahead of them, which only serves to make the issue more emotional. The process required to complete this type of search can result in the adoptee's becoming obsessed with the endeavor. Birthparents also initiate searches and reunions.

Although agencies have established registries across North America, each province and state varies in its policies and procedures. Registries operate by the voluntary registration of the adoptee and of the birthparent. The adoptee must have attained the age of majority to register and receive information. If both names match, the information is exchanged—often through a third party. In some places, the adopting parents must consent to this process. In other places, adoptees have access to their original birth records when they reach the age of majority.

Adoption agencies are receiving an increasing number of requests for information from adopted children and birthparents. Over the years, adoption agencies have had difficulty in deciding on the extent of background information to be given to the adoptive family and how much of this should be shared with the child.

Adoptive parents may feel threatened by their adopted children's questions about policies on confidentiality and by questions about their birthparents. If you place your child for adoption, however, you will need to remember that once the child is accepted into the home of the adoptive family, it is the love and the relationship that develops that makes the child their son or daughter. You do not need a blood tie to love someone very deeply. Adoptive parents can often become the forgotten party in the adoption triangle. No one seems to take on the role of providing them with support over the years to help them deal with their child's questions and feelings about his or her other parents. Adoptive parents will need support to help them feel secure in their role as parents with increased openness in adoption. All three parties in the adoption triangle, as well as all the professionals involved, need to have comfort with this open attitude if it is to have positive effects.

If you are placing a child for adoption now, you will need to evaluate how open you plan to be with people in the future about your pregnancy. Will you be open with your relatives, friends, and neighbors? What about future boyfriends? How might you deal with the appearance of a child on your doorstep years later? In these times, it could very well become a reality. If this should happen, the adoptee may be more prepared for this step then you because he or she has been thinking about and working toward this for some time during the search. You might be totally unprepared and may have even kept your pregnancy a secret from people who came into your life after the birth of this child. If you are honest and open about your pregnancy with significant people in your life, you could prevent problems later.

When your child becomes an adult, you may choose to place your name on a registry, if one exists in your area. This might give you some consolation that if your child should feel a strong need to know about you, he or she can have access to this information. It can provide you with a means of passing on an explanation of the circumstances of the adoption. It may put your mind a rest knowing that your child is okay after all these years and may put your child's mind at rest once background gaps are filled in.

Accounts by three other people who are also members of lifelong adoption triangles follow. They have all thought about this issue and have generously shared their thoughts and feelings. Their stories are not intended to portray a particular bias for or against adoption, but rather to offer you a variety of personal experiences.

Linda

Linda is 41 years of age. She is married and has three children. She is an adult adoptee who has completed a search to find her birthparents. She is now actively engaged in work with an organization that helps adult adoptees locate their birthparents. Linda also assists parents who have relinquished children for adoption by placing their names on the voluntary registry. Linda shares her adoption experiences in the hope that this may assist teenagers who are considering placing their babies for adoption gain insight into the lifelong consequences of adoption.

When I was 4 years old, I was told that I was adopted. I didn't completely understand what adoption meant, but after being told, I was curious. I asked my mother many questions about my biological mother. I asked what she looked like, what the circumstances were, and why she had given me up for adoption. I was told that she was a married woman and that she died after giving birth to me. My father was apparently unable to keep me as there was another child. He was financially unable to look after me. I was therefore put up for adoption.

Of course, my curiosity continued and periodically I would ask questions in reference to her. I asked my mother what my original name was. My mother seemed to be very honest with me. She didn't show any signs of being uncomfortable with the situation. I have an adopted brother, and he didn't seem to have the same degree of curiosity about his natural parents as I had about mine. At times I even asked about his adoption.

My questions were not continuous. The topic would just come up. Other children would mention it, and then when they found out that I was adopted, I would get the old comments such as, "Your mother didn't want you." I remember going home one day heartbroken and relating the incident to my mother. She said, "Well, never mind. You tell them that when their mothers had them, they had to take what they got. We were able to choose you." I found that consoling.

When I was told by my parents that I was adopted, they said that they had been called by social services and told that they had a little girl. They said that they went to the agency and picked me out of all these lovely babies in rows and rows of cribs. I thought it was wonderful. I was told that my feet were deformed and that they had turned upward. When my adoptive mother saw this, she was afraid to mention it to my adoptive father because she thought that he might not want me.

As I reached my teenage years, I became more curious and particularly so when I got married at age 16. Soon after my marriage, I gave birth to a child, and the desire to know about my biological family became more intense. Then I was concerned not only about myself but also about this other little human being. I had to pass on something to this child, such as background information, medical information, and information about physical characteristics.

These questions came to my mind when I went into the hospital to have my first child. I could relate to what it must have been like for my natural mother to give birth to me. My natural mother would have been 19 when I was born. There wasn't that much difference in age between us at the time we first gave birth.

I was terrified when I was taken into the delivery room because I'd been told about my natural mother's apparent death after childbirth. All these thoughts flashed back in my mind. I was quite convinced that I would die after delivery. Here I was 16 years old, and I was so naïve and stupid when it came to childbirth. I hadn't been able to talk with my adoptive mother about giving birth because I felt that she wouldn't have any idea about what to expect, as she had never given birth to a child. I didn't attend prenatal classes because they weren't as prevalent back then. I really didn't have a clue about what to expect.

I was still a teenager during this pregnancy and marriage. I was still growing up. I had to deal with all of that at the time as well as thinking about my own mother and all my fears related to childbirth.

As I was adopted, I couldn't imagine myself being born. I somehow couldn't relate to being carried in my mother's womb for nine months, or my mother being in a delivery room giving birth. I felt as if all of a sudden I was here on this earth, and I didn't know how I got here. I knew how birth happened, but it was as if I had just appeared like an alien from outer space.

My curiosity about my biological parents began to blossom when I had children of my own. Years later I heard a program on the radio. On this program, there were two adoptees discussing their experiences and thoughts about being adopted and their searches to find their biological parents. I could really relate to this. It was quite a revelation to me because I'd never been able to talk with anybody else who had been adopted. I thought, my goodness, there are actually other people out there with the same thoughts and same desires as I have.

I thought that I was not the Lone Ranger after all. It took me a couple of weeks to work up my nerve though, to finally phone the number that was given over the radio. I didn't know what to expect on the other end of the phone. As it turned out, the girl who answered the phone was also adopted. So I began relating all of my feelings to her, and she actually knew what I was talking about. From then on, I started to search for my natural parents. I was told where to write for my nonidentifying background information. I was fortunate enough to know the name given to me at birth to assist me in my search. My adoptive parents had their own lawyer draw up the adoption papers, so they had access to my original name. I was told this name by my mother and kept it written down. Once I received my background information, it was a matter of doing a lot of research, writing a lot of letters, going through directory pages, and making fishing phone calls.

It took me approximately a year before I finally made the initial contact with my natural mother. The first contact was made through an intermediary. This third person phoned my natural mother and made a few basic inquiries about my birth date and name. As soon as she said yes, the information was correct, she immediately wanted to speak to me. I got on the phone, and she was crying. It was a very emotional experience. She told me that on that very day she had been out in the yard thinking about me.

This year of searching had been very intense. I became obsessed with the search. I don't think anything could have stopped me. I was a proverbial pain to friends and family. All I could talk about was this search. Once the search was completed, it was less than a month before I actually met my real mother. Her family met us at the airport, and it was a very emotional scene. It was more emotional for her as she had kept me for six months before giving me up for adoption. She had actually breastfed me. I didn't know her, but she had memories of me as a very tiny baby. She kept referring to me as "my baby." This was hard for me to deal with. There were many questions, looks, touches, and conversations.

Suddenly it was as if I was part of the human race. Now I can actually say that I know where my mother is. I know where I inherit certain traits and why I look like this. After the reunion, there is a period of coming down after the intense high feeling. I went through periods when I did not get a letter, and I would wonder if she had changed her mind. I felt up and down for a while. Apparently she experienced the same process. I actually went into a state of depression afterward. I had such a tremendously good feeling, and then all of a sudden I was back to reality and had to deal with everyday occurrences. I had to integrate this experience into my present life. I had to sort out how I was going to relate to this person who had given birth to me.

The most supportive people were the volunteers in the adoptees organization. Most of these volunteers had experienced a reunion themselves and knew what to expect. I really advise an adoptee doing a search to be affiliated with an organization for moral support. It is a heavy undertaking to live through. In preparation for a search you have to think specifically about what you might come up against. It is not like a soap opera where everyone runs across a field with outstretched arms. You have to be able to accept rejection. The mother might say that this is a part of her life that she would rather forget. I know that deep down natural mothers never really forget, but they just don't want to deal with it. You also have to be prepared for the fact that the person might be deceased or that the woman didn't tell her husband. The relationship has to be on her terms.

You become a different person after the reunion. My natural mother was not as prepared as I was for the reunion. If she had been registered, then she would have decided that was what she wanted and would have expected it could happen. I had a whole year while I was working on my search to prepare for the reunion. In her mind, she had wished it might happen but never really thought that it would. The phone call from me came out of the blue for her. It was like her fantasy turned into reality. Often when she would see a little girl who might have been my age, and especially if she found that the child was adopted, she wondered if this girl was her child. She didn't know that I had moved to another province. She just took it for granted that because I was born in Ontario my adopted parents remained there.

Both of my adoptive parents were deceased when I began my search. I would still have gone through with my search even if they had been alive. I don't feel that they would have felt hurt because when I think back to the times when I asked questions about my natural parents, my adoptive parents had no inhibitions. They were not reluctant to answer my questions. Children have a way of picking up on their parent's feelings. I did not sense any signs of uncomfortableness or disapproval from my parents.

After I found out that my real mother was still alive, I realized that the information I had been given was not true. My natural mother had not died. The only way I can think to explain this is possibly by the fact that my adoptive parents were given the background information verbally by the social worker rather than having it in written form. This allowed for misinterpretation. When I received my background information during my search, it stated that my natural mother's mother had died during childbirth, so possibly my adoptive mother got this information mixed up over the years. Details may have been forgotten over time.

But by growing up with the misinformation, I carried that fear about childbirth through all my pregnancies. The fear is still there in my subconscious, and it is pretty hard to shake it loose.

Overall, the search and reunion were worthwhile to me. I now know whom I look like. All of my questions are finally answered. There was only one person who could answer those questions for me, and that was the woman who gave birth to me. She was the one who told me what day I was born, what time of the night, and after how many hours of labor. These were all things that I could never imagine. Finally I know, and I can relax. I am at peace with myself and no longer wondering. It is as though I had awakened from a state of amnesia.

Now I work with an adoptees reform organization, and I am able to help others. I think that it would be helpful in the adoption process if natural mothers were given more information about the adopting families. Recently, one woman told me that her child was born prematurely. She didn't get to see her child before the adoption. She didn't know if the child was alive or dead. When I tell natural mothers that they are entitled to nonidentifying information about the adoptive family, it's as though I had just given them a million dollars.

I don't think the natural mothers were really given any options. Many of the women I have spoken with were just told that they were going to have to give their babies up for adoption. There were not as many options a number of years ago as there are today. There were not as many resources to help girls who became pregnant.

Many of the women I have had contact with felt pressure from social workers to place their children for adoption. They were told to get on with their lives and just forget about it. From what I have observed, I conclude that it just doesn't happen that way. They can't give a part of themselves and forget that it has ever happened. Most natural mothers say to me, "If only I had known." I feel so helpless when I'm talking to them. Usually I try to put them in touch with another mother in our organization who has had more time to deal with the situation. Sometimes it can be helpful for them to talk with somebody else who has gone through a similar experience. So many of these women are unable to even discuss the adoption with their closest friends because "good girls" don't get pregnant. The fact that they register with our organization gives them a sense that they are doing something purposeful.

Our organization does as much as it can for parents who have given up their children. We have offered our facilities to them to hold meetings in if they so choose. We try to get them to participate and to help them feel that they are contributing to something worthwhile.

If a teenager decides to place her baby for adoption, I would like to suggest that she consider writing a letter to the child. She could express how she felt at the time of the adoption and possibly the reasons why or add a gift that she might want to pass on to the child. Something in the mother's own handwriting might mean a great deal to the child later on. These articles can be passed on to the child as long as the adoptive parents accept them. It is my experience these days that the adoptive parents often do accept such items as long as there is no identifying information about the natural parents.

Bruce

Bruce is an adoptive parent who shares with us his own experience in adopting two children. He comments on issues related to adoption from his own perspective. He is 44 years old and is the director of social work at a children's hospital. His two adopted children are Elizabeth, who is 6 and a half years old, and Rosemary, who is 3 and a half.

Both adoptions were very stirring. I remember them vividly. When you go through the process of trying to adopt a child, there is a waiting period. My wife and I waited about nine months for Elizabeth. Then we received the phone call, which came out of the blue. The call came on Monday while I was at work. It was so very exciting. Of course, the agency wanted me to come down the next day to get information. I phoned my wife, Lou. They gave me a little information over the phone about Elizabeth's background and said that she was French Canadian. I can remember leaving work very excited and wondering what name we might give her. All sorts of thoughts went through my mind. One thing I remember clearly is that I had a tape of a French singer in my car. I played this tape on the way home as I thought of her French background.

This is the way in which we had our children. We didn't have the birth experience, but it was exciting, with all the pounding blood and high-energy feeling. Lou rushed home, and of course we went over all the details again. The next day we went to the child welfare agency to receive more information about the baby's background.

Background information is important to have as an adoptive parent because the children will need to know later on. Already Elizabeth, at age 6, is starting to ask more questions about her adoption. She first asked questions about adoption when we introduced the word to her at about age 3. One time Elizabeth said to Lou, "I came out of your tummy." Lou explained that she hadn't come out of her tummy but had come out of another lady's tummy. Lou told her that it had not been possible for Elizabeth to remain with her natural mother as there was no dad. Lou didn't go into great detail but said that we very much wanted to have a baby, and it worked out that we were able to have her, so we became her parents. I was in the garden painting that summer when Elizabeth approached me after talking with Lou. Elizabeth said that she was in this tummy and really wanted to get out of the tummy and get going. She said, "And you wanted a baby, so I was your baby." Elizabeth seemed to feel a sense of belonging.

Sometimes adopted children feel that they start their life off by being rejected, when there was never any sense of rejection. I remember when we went to get Elizabeth at the hospital. We went into the nursery, and my wife bundled her up. I remember us both sitting on the plane coming home just staring down at Elizabeth. She was a beautiful baby. We felt such acceptance.

Sometimes adopted children feel as if they are not as good as other children, or they put themselves down because they feel there is a difference. I think everyone has something different in their life. Adoption entails a set of circumstances which happens to some people. But it can be seen in that light as a difference rather than as a rejection. Giving a baby up for adoption is a decision based on a set of circumstances.

I think of my girls as tremendously special children. I am thankful and grateful to the natural parents. My wife and I are beneficiaries. I remember my neighbor's having mentioned to me that both girls are very pretty. He wondered how their mothers ever gave them up for adoption. I told him that there were circumstances and that life isn't easy. If it hadn't happened, we wouldn't have had the children. So it has been beneficial to us.

To comment on the gradual liberalization of policies with regard to confidentiality in adoption, I would like to mention that Lou and I have talked about this. If our children should have the desire for further information or ever want the opportunity to meet their natural parents, we would be quite supportive. We do not feel that it is a problem. About a month ago, Elizabeth asked Lou if she would ever be able to find her real mother. Lou said that she was her mother now, but that she may be able to find her biological mother when she grows up. That seemed to satisfy Elizabeth for the moment.

Many adoptive parents feel threatened by their children's questions about their natural parents. But the whole business of being a parent is based on the relationship that you have with your child, regardless of whether that child is adopted or naturally born to you. If you have a good relationship with your child, that is the really important element. If everything has gone well for 16 or 17 years, that is not all going to go away suddenly because the child wants to have some sense of her own roots. This desire is very natural. As a parent I worry that it could be painful, and part of me would like to protect my children from pain. But very quickly I realize that this is impossible. If something is really important to Elizabeth or Rosemary, and I really care about them, then it would be a rejection if I said, "No. You can't do that." That would be ridiculous if it were important to them.

I think that Lou and I are prepared for these issues to arise. We expect that our children may very well have these desires. I imagine that they have very nice natural parents. I have some sense of them from the history. I don't think that I would have any negative feelings toward these people at all.

There is a lot of criticism about the adoption process. Some people who want to adopt a child and are turned down may feel disenchanted with the system, but I feel that adoption is a very serious business and should not be taken lightly. I think that parenting is serious and whoever takes on the role needs to think about it. Before you adopt a child you are forced to look at becoming a parent. You make a choice to be a parent. I think that is good, and I wouldn't want the process to be different.

Some of the questions that you are asked by the social workers at the child welfare agency are a bit difficult, such as how you handle a child who says, "I don't have to do that! I'm not your child anyway." I can remember being asked that question. Most of all, you have to be comfortable with all the issues that might arise with an adopted child. You need to be comfortable in your role as an adoptive parent. If you feel that it is your second choice, then this feeling will get transmitted to the child in some manner. The child will feel as if he or she is second best. I think that you really have to look at your own feelings and your acceptance of being an adoptive parent. There will be issues that will arise with adopted children that will not come up with children who are naturally born to you.

It is very important that adopted children grow up with a feeling that being adopted is okay. There is nothing wrong with being an adopted child. Openness about the adoption should be encouraged. In fact, an example comes to mind concerning our babysitter. When Elizabeth was about 3 years old, the babysitter said, "We will have to be careful about using the word 'adoption.'" I replied, "Why would we? We've always been open with Elizabeth." Only recently did Elizabeth tell the babysitter that she was adopted. It seemed to be a relief for the babysitter to have that out in the open. Often children can be more comfortable with issues than adults can.

Suzanne

Suzanne is 37 years old. She is married and has two children, ages 16 and 4. She is a board member at an adoptees organization. Suzanne is an adult adoptee and also the birthmother of a baby born when she was a teenager whom she gave up for adoption. Suzanne shares her experiences with us from this dual perspective.

I knew from a very young age that I was adopted. I always wanted to know who my biological parents were. I learned that this was a subject that was not to be discussed too deeply with my adoptive mother. She would always say, "I am your mother." When I was 12 years old, my parents did tell me my name at birth. They had met my natural mother and they had the adoption order in their possession. My natural mother had kept me for a month before placing me for adoption. My parents had heard that there was a pregnant woman who lived in the same neighborhood as my grandmother. This woman was planning to give up her baby for adoption, and my parents wanted a child. The adoption was largely arranged privately, but the Children's Aid Society was involved in the process.

As I was growing up, my dad's family would always refer to me as "adopted." I felt very left out. My sister and I felt excluded because we were both adopted, and the relatives made us feel that we were not really one of them. Even in a large group of people including aunts, uncles, and cousins, we still did not have a sense of belonging. Now I refuse to see my father's relatives.

My adoptive parents were told that my natural mother was going back to Alberta to complete school and become a nurse. When I gave birth to my first child, I can remember being in the hospital, and I wondered if one of these nurses might be my mother. In fact, every time I was in the hospital I thought this. It's strange.

Three years ago, I was in a drugstore and saw the book *Adopted.* I almost broke my neck getting down the aisle to reach it. I flipped through the pages and saw the address and phone number for Parent Finders. I wrote this number down and went home to think about it. I thought about phoning this organization for about a month. I was afraid and nervous. I didn't know who might be on the other end of the line, but there was really no way that they could know who I was. I was afraid that my adoptive father would find out. I thought that it would be too much for him, as he was 71 years old. At this time, my adoptive mother was no longer alive.

My father didn't know about my search for my natural mother until after I'd completed it. I thought that there was no reason upsetting him in case I was never able to find her. I decided that I would tell him if I found her.

It took me a year to find her and after I did, I told my dad. When I told him, I was really upset. I was crying and told him that it didn't mean that I didn't love him. I told him that I'd done something and that I'd done it for myself. First of all, he thought that I was dying. Then I told him that I'd started a search for my natural mother and I'd found her. He told me that he always thought I'd do something like that. He knew that I'd always asked questions about my background. I wondered why he had never talked about it with me because I learned that he had known my mother's name and many other things. It would have taken me far less time to find her if I'd spoken with him first.

My dad didn't react the way I thought he was going to. He just asked me why I hadn't come to him. He was very understanding. We talked about it for quite a while, and he asked me if I was going to meet her. I told him that I likely would and that I'd only talked with her on the phone so far. He said that he'd like to meet her again. This surprised me. I just stared at him and asked why he had never said anything to me about her. He hadn't been sure how to approach the subject. He hadn't wanted to make me feel hurt or rejected. I thought, "This is beautiful. Here we are both trying so hard to protect each other from hurt." I couldn't believe it.

The day that I found out where my natural mother was, I had an intermediary call her. Since then, I have been in contact with her, and my present relationship with her could be described as a distant friendship. She still feels guilty after all these years. She feels guilty about having given me up for adoption and for the fact she doesn't love me the way that she loves her other three children. She had not told her husband about her pregnancy before their marriage so he does not know about my existence in her life now. When I have visited their home, I have been introduced as their daughter's friend. That makes me feel awkward.

When I began to search, I didn't go looking for a mother. I went looking for where I had come from, who I am, and why I do the things I do. I was interested in where I had inherited certain traits. I wanted to know my medical history. I wondered if I had any half-brothers or half-sisters. I did actually meet my half-sister, and we now get along really well.

My adoptive mother and I did not have a very good relationship. But when somebody refers to my mother, I relate to my adopted mother and not to my natural mother. My natural mother is the woman who gave birth to me. I have a lot of her characteristics and some of her personality traits. This may sound very cold, but that is how it is. She doesn't know me. When I met her it was not a magical event. It was reality.

I can also look at this issue from the other angle of having given a baby up for adoption when I was a teenager. My daughter would now be 18 years old. She will reach the age of majority next year. I don't really think that I will choose to look for her, although part of me would like to look for her. It's virtually impossible to start a search unless I have a name to begin with. The only name I would have would be the name I gave her at birth. I don't know her adopted name. The information I have on her adoptive family is very brief and sketchy. It could apply to any one of a million people. I don't know if she has ever been told that she is adopted. If she has been told, I don't think that I have the right to go looking for her even though she is my flesh and blood. I feel that it is up to her to make these decisions. If she wants to know where she comes from then that is her decision. I will make myself available to her in any way that I can just to let her know that I'm here if she ever wants to meet me or talk with me. I'd like to have a good relationship with her, but it would not be a mother/daughter relationship. It would probably take a long time to establish any type of relationship.

When I think back about the contact with my natural mother, I realize that she was totally unprepared for my phone call. I had people to talk with through the organization who had been through similar experiences. They understood what I felt. I have this group behind me who would be there to support me if my daughter located me. I think that I would be able to cope with it in a much better manner than my natural mother was able to. My family is aware of the situation so I don't have the guilt about hiding anything.

At the same time, I can't get too psyched up about it. My daughter may never phone me, or she could call out of the blue at any time. She could call me next year when she becomes an adult, or she could call me when she is 40 years old. It could happen tomorrow, or it may never happen. That makes it very hard to prepare for. I can only anticipate that it might happen to me. I would feel lucky if she does want to know about her roots. I would like to know if she is alive, if she is healthy, if she is happy. I hope she's had a good life.

I can honestly say that I gave my daughter up for adoption out of necessity. There was just no other way at the time. I didn't realize that possibly I could have found a job. I didn't realize that I could have lived on welfare. I played the role of the obedient adoptee and did what my mom said. My mother said, "You are going to give the baby up for adoption. You can't go out and get a place to live. You can't get a job to support yourself and a child. Who's going to hire you and take you in?" I really believed that if I showed my face everybody would know what a bad girl I was and that would be it. I remember walking down the street and running into a friend from school about a month after I'd had the child. This friend looked shocked. I hadn't seen her for about a year. I thought, "She knows."

I grew up in Vancouver, but I moved to a small community. I was in the last months of the 12th grade when I found out that I was pregnant. I was 19 years old, and my boyfriend was the same age. We wanted to get married. My parents didn't want me to marry him, and his parents didn't want him to marry me. The prospect of living together was out of the question. At the time it was more socially acceptable to be pregnant and not married than pregnant and living with my boyfriend.

While I was pregnant, my mother dragged me around with her to visit her friends and paraded me to church each week. It was as though I were part of the cross that she had to bear. She was showing everyone that this is what happens when you adopt because you don't know what you're getting. My mom would imply that it was probably my "bad blood" that had led to my pregnancy. I was made to feel very ashamed and embarrassed about my pregnancy. I figured that this pregnancy had to be the worst thing that could happen to me. My mother wouldn't have let me consider abortion. She felt that I had made my bed so I had to lie in it and go to term with the pregnancy.

The first time I went to the doctor to see if I was pregnant, my mom let me go by myself. From then on, she went with me on every visit. She insisted on being in the examination room with me each time. She would talk with the doctor as though I weren't even there. At one point she talked to the doctor about putting me into a home for unwed mothers. She felt that I was an embarrassment, and it would be like a punishment for me. One of her favorite lines was, "We had to do such and such with Suzanne. We had to ground her, or we had to put her into a home for unwed mothers." The pregnancy was seen as just another thing that I had done to her. It took until the last couple of years for me to realize that I had bent over backwards to please my mom. I had worn myself out trying to deserve a word of acceptance from her. I wanted her to tell me that I had done something that made her proud, but she never did.

I sit here now and look at myself and think about how I've been a fool to accept her concept of me. I had gone to such lengths to try to gain her approval. My adoptive father was the exact opposite. I got along with my dad really well. After a while, my mom's words began to have an effect on me and I began to believe that I became pregnant just to upset her. When I look back now I realize that I didn't get pregnant to aggravate her.

I was very ignorant as far as sex education was concerned. My mother could never have children, and I wasn't around many pregnant women. Pregnant was a word that had little meaning to me. I couldn't visualize a pregnant woman. I realized that I was missing my periods. I didn't want to admit to myself that I was pregnant. I started getting morning sickness, and I began to worry. When the doctor confirmed my pregnancy, I realized that I really was pregnant. I understood how I became pregnant, but I had never thought that it would happen to me. I thought that I was basically quite good, and it was only bad girls who became pregnant. I figured that I was not bad, so how could I possibly get pregnant?

I really didn't feel that I had any options regarding my pregnancy. My mother told me that I would never bring the child into her house. The social worker, the doctor, my parents, and my boyfriend's parents convinced me that I'd never find a job and could not cope with life if I kept the baby. I felt overwhelmed. No one said anything at all positive. The most positive comment anyone made during my whole pregnancy was that I was healthy. I might have decided to place my baby for adoption anyway, if my parents had let me make the choice myself. If they had asked me what I really wanted to do and allowed me to arrive at my own decision, I think that I'd be a lot less bitter today. It seemed that this baby was the first person in my whole life who was my own flesh and blood, and I felt pressure to give her away.

Now my adoptive mother is dead. My boyfriend's adoptive father is dead. Of these two families, my father and my boyfriend's adoptive mother remain alive and still reside in the same small community. My boyfriend's mother and my mother really went at me during my pregnancy. They ganged up on me. The fathers were in the background, passively supporting their wives. Now my father had the nerve to ask if I'm doing anything about finding his grandchild. My boyfriend's mother is saying the same thing. I find this very hard to deal with.

It took me a long time to regain my self-confidence. It was actually only about three years ago when I joined the Adoptees Reform Group that I was able to find the confidence to talk with people about these personal subjects. I was into my 30s by this time.

My present husband and I talked about my pregnancy before we were married. The topic came up in a discussion with friends. It didn't seem to bother him one way or the other. I was a little bit hesitant about telling him, but I was only going out with him at the time. I thought that if this scared him away then he was not worth having in my life. Everybody has a skeleton in the family closet.

When I discussed my pregnancy with my first husband, it turned out that he had fathered a child before we were married. It was as if we confessed to each other. The topic was never brought up again, but we didn't stay together long.

My eldest daughter is now 16. I told her about my pregnancy when she was almost 15. Since I am a member of an adoptees reform group, I can't see myself creeping around whispering. She would probably figure it out anyway. I wanted to tell her for a couple of reasons. First of all, she is a girl. The same thing could very easily happen to her. I wanted her to know that if she did become pregnant, she could tell me. I would want her to be able to come and talk with me about it. I was really afraid to tell her because I feared that she would judge me. I thought that she might be appalled that her mother had had a child out of wedlock, and that she had given the baby away. But my daughter was very understanding. She was thrilled at the fact that she has an older sister somewhere. I seemed to be more human to her after I told her. Even mom isn't perfect. I felt it was important that my family hear the facts from me and not from someone else. It was important to me to be open and honest with my family. This would help to prepare them in case my daughter ever comes looking for me.

At the time of my pregnancy, I was told that I would forget about the whole thing and would carry on with my life. I did carry on, but I didn't forget. You can hardly forget the pregnancy, the birth, and the adoption. I wasn't allowed to see my child in the hospital. The nurses, the doctors, the social worker, and my family wouldn't let me see my baby. They said that it would be harder for me to give the child up for adoption. I don't agree with that. I felt that I had the right to see my baby. I remember walking down the hall to the nursery and looking in the window to see my baby. I knew which baby was mine because she was the one who was farthest away from the window. I can remember seeing her dark head. Everyone I asked to see the baby felt that it was better that I didn't and felt that I would probably forget. I would recommend that a teenager see her child before she signs the final adoption papers. I think that would make it more of a reality. Some people say that all babies look alike, but they don't. If you actually hold a child, you will think about your decision more seriously.

When I gave birth to my other two children, I found that it evoked these past feelings. Even with my last pregnancy, it brought back memories. I feel sorry for my eldest girl because it is like she almost has had to be two children to me. She had to be the first and second. I probably expected a lot from her because I gave the first baby up for adoption. With my eldest daughter, I felt very possessive—that this was my baby.

During my pregnancy as a teenager I didn't have anyone as a support. I was allowed to see my boyfriend for a while. Then my parents would not allow me to see him. I felt that I had brought this whole thing on myself, and I had to pay the price. I tried to block out my thoughts. After the child was born, I remember talking to a good friend of mine. I just decided to phone and talk with her. It was really strange. We sat there and hemmed and hawed. We both wanted someone to talk with but were afraid of the other's reaction. As it turned out, she had had a baby whom she had given up for adoption a month before I had. We realized that we could have been together through the whole process. We could have sat, talked, and cried together. So I found somebody after the pregnancy. I could have kicked myself for not having called her before.

I lost contact with my friends during this period. I was convinced that I was bad and that no one would want to have anything to do with me. I felt that I couldn't take any more rejection, so I stayed away from my friends.

If I had the opportunity to talk with teenagers who are pregnant now I would tell them to do what they want to do. Find out what you want. Do what you feel is best for you, not what your parents want. This is a very personal decision that only you can make. You are the one who will have to live with the decision. You should take everything into consideration and search out all options.

Appendix D

Website Resources and Phone Contacts

Crisis Phone Line
Child Help Hotline (USA)
800/422-4453 (free call in the United States)

Pregnancy
Unsure About Your Pregnancy Booklet Online
www.cbctrust.com/unsure.html

Pregnancy Options Workbook Online
www.gynpages.com/workbook

Healthy Teen Network
www.healthyteennetwork.org

Birth Control and Abortion Information
Planned Parenthood USA
800/230-PLAN (free call)
www.plannedparenthood.org

Planned Parenthood Canada
www.ppfc.ca

Birth Control
www.ultimatebirthcontrol.com

Abortion Information and Clinic Directories
www.abortionclinic.org
www.gynpages.com
www.morgentaler.ca

National Abortion Federation
www.prochoice.org
Hotline: 800/772-9100 (English and Spanish—free call)

Adoption

National Adoption Information Clearinghouse—lists licensed
adoption agencies in the United States
703/352-3488
www.calib.com/naic

Canadian Adoption Information
www.adoption.ca

Teen Parenting
www.girlmom.com
www.kidsrights.com/teen_parenting.asp

STDs

www.iwannaknow.org

About the Author

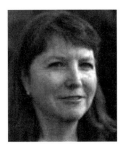

Patricia Roles, MSW, RSW, BCATR, is a social worker and birthmother who relinquished a baby for adoption as a teenager. She was born in England, raised in Ontario, and now resides in Vancouver, British Columbia. She obtained her social service certificate and bachelor's degree in social work from Ryerson University, her master's degree in social work from the University of British Columbia, and her postgraduate certificate in art therapy from the BC School of Art Therapy. Her background includes both adult and child psychiatry; counseling with children, youth, and families with chronic and acute illness; and eating disorders. She has facilitated counseling groups for birthparents through family services. She works at BC Children's Hospital as a family therapist in the eating disorders program and as a clinical supervisor in the social work department. She also has a private e-counseling practice through her website at www.e-mailtherapy.com.

Other publications by Patricia Roles through the Child Welfare League of America include *Saying Goodbye to a Baby, Volume 1: The Birth Parent's Guide to Loss and Grief in Adoption* (1989) and *Saying Goodbye to a Baby, Volume 2: A Counselor's Guide to Birth Parent Loss and Grief in Adoption* (1989).